Sickening

Sickening

ANTI-BLACK RACISM AND HEALTH DISPARITIES IN THE UNITED STATES

Anne Pollock

UNIVERSITY OF MINNESOTA PRESS
Minneapolis
London

Portions of chapter 3 are adapted from "On the Suspended Sentences of the Scott Sisters: Mass Incarceration, Kidney Donation, and the Biopolitics of Race in the United States," *Science, Technology, and Human Values* 40, no. 2 (2015): 250–71.

Published by the University of Minnesota Press
111 Third Avenue South, Suite 290
Minneapolis, MN 55401-2520
http://www.upress.umn.edu

ISBN 978-1-5179-1171-3 (hc)
ISBN 978-1-5179-1172-0 (pb)

A Cataloging-in-Publication record for this book is available from the Library of Congress.

UMP LSI

Contents

Acknowledgments   vii

Introduction   1

1. Terrorism: The Deaths of Black Postal Workers
in the 2001 Anthrax Attacks   21

2. Un/natural Disaster: Chronic Disease
after Hurricane Katrina   43

3. Mass Incarceration: On the Suspended Sentences
of the Scott Sisters   61

4. Environmental Racism: Protecting GM's Machines
While Abandoning Flint's People   79

5. Police Brutality: Enforcing Segregation
at a Pool Party   95

6. Reproductive Injustice:
Serena Williams's Birth Story   117

Conclusion   133

Notes   147

Index   191

Acknowledgments

I am deeply grateful to the American Council of Learned Societies, which awarded me a fellowship that gave me the time and space to complete the full draft of the manuscript.

This project developed over many years and has benefited from the support of my academic homes: MIT, where I began my PhD in September 2001 and first started serious academic exploration of many of these topics in racism and health, first in classes with Evelynn Hammonds and Ken Manning and later with support from the Center for the Study of Diversity in Science, Technology, and Medicine under the leadership of David Jones; Georgia Tech, where I served on the faculty for ten years, learning from colleagues in the CDC Working Group on Racism and Health and later in the cross-institutional Working Group on Race and Racism in Contemporary Biomedicine, and learning from students whom I taught in courses including Biomedicine and Culture and Science, Technology, and Race; and finally, my current home, the Department of Global Health and Social Medicine at King's College London, which provided a Seed Grant that allowed me to benefit from Beauty Dhlamini's insightful research assistance for chapter 6 and more broadly has provided an incomparable intellectual environment in which to explore questions of health, medicine, and society. While I was preparing the revised manuscript under lockdown, Katherine Behar provided critical help with the images. The University of Minnesota Press has provided invaluable support for bringing the project to fruition as a book, especially Jason Weidemann and Zenyse Miller.

Many chapters began as conference presentations at the Society for Social Studies of Science and benefited from engagement with the audiences there. I also had the chance to present an individual chapter at the

University of Amsterdam Department of Anthropology's Ir/relevance of Race in Science and Society seminar series, and an overview of the book as a whole at both my own Department of Global Health and Social Medicine Seminar at King's College London and the STS Circle at Harvard University.

Numerous colleagues and friends generously gave feedback on various iterations of chapters in progress, including Ruha Benjamin, Rasmus Birk, Silvia Camporesi, Carol Colatrella, Philip Cohen, Joe Dumit, Faith Groesbeck, Jennifer Hamilton, Tony Hatch, Amy Hinterberger, David Jones, Katrina Karkazis, Emma Kowal, Amade M'charek, Susana Morris, Alondra Nelson, Michelle Pentecost, Thao Phan, Manu Platt, Amy Slaton, Lindsay Smith, Brett St Louis, Judith Suissa, Siggie Vertommen, Kate Weiner, Lewis Wheaton, and Ros Williams. Sarah Blacker, Madeleine Pape, and Natali Valdez each taught from the draft manuscript in their undergraduate classes, and they and their students provided additional layers of insight. I owe a special thanks to Amy Agigian and Dartricia Rollins, who provided comments on the full manuscript. An extra measure of gratitude goes to my writing group—Mary McDonald, Nassim Parvin, and Jennifer Singh—who have remained treasured friends and intellectual interlocutors even though I left our beloved Atlanta and who provided generous feedback on many iterations.

Finally, Maital Dar has been a true partner not only in life but also in this work: she has often been my first interlocutor as the events occurred, has helped me to prepare the conference papers in which most of the chapters originated, and has been an invaluable editor as I completed the book. I cannot possibly thank her enough.

Introduction

London, July 4, 2020

In spring 2020, when so many people all over the world first became transfixed by the dangers of the novel coronavirus that causes COVID-19, there was a strong narrative that we were "all in this together" as we were implored to "flatten the curve." This message was pervasive in the United States, where I am from, and in the United Kingdom, where I live—filling my newsfeed of both mainstream media and social media. And yet, with each passing week, the racially and ethnically unequal pattern of who was most likely to be sickened and killed by COVID-19 became increasingly visible. If the looming curve looked mathematical and indiscriminate, that obscured the very different lived experiences that structure epidemiological risk.

As spring turned to summer, high-profile incidents of deadly violence against Black people sparked an awakening from COVID's numbing numbers: the vigilante killing of jogger Ahmaud Arbery, the police killing of Breonna Taylor in her own home, and especially the police murder of George Floyd caught on video footage that has been widely shared. These murders and the righteous protests that they have sparked remind us that, in our racist societies, unequal vulnerability is not new.

These crises of COVID-19 and of police brutality can call our attention to the factors that contribute to health inequality, such as systems of health care and of policing, in a context of segregated neighborhoods and unequal urban infrastructures. They also point toward the depth of the societal transformation that would be required for Black Lives to be treated as if they truly Matter.

The deaths from COVID-19 and the recent police and vigilante murders are acute instances of chronic health and social inequalities. And the sources of these inequalities far exceed the institutions of health care and policing, extending to the broader social, political, and economic structures that shape unequal lived experiences.

During this disrupted period, as the news cycle and social media cycle both churn relentlessly, it can feel hard to keep up. Going against the rush to take time for considered analysis is not the default setting of social media engagement. The speed of the onslaught of information on social media is part of its design. Consider: Facebook's original corporate motto was "move fast and break things," and this kind of recklessness has been a pervasive mind-set among tech companies. Yet, as Black feminist analyst of science and technology Ruha Benjamin points out, that approach has included a disregard for breaking *people*.[1] Benjamin insists that technology design and use—including social media—should instead "move slower and protect people,"[2] and I would add that the same is true for the way that we engage with media images and stories more broadly. If we take the time to sit with these events, take them in, and both unpack their specificities and attend to how they are part of broader structures, they can become concrete entry points into understanding the wide-ranging ways in which racism operates.

It is in this spirit—simultaneously urgent and slow—that I sit down to complete this book.

Sickening: Anti-Black Racism and Health Disparities in the United States explores a series of distinct, evocative events to illuminate wide-ranging aspects of racial health disparities in the contemporary United States. I start at a time before the widespread use of social media, in the immediate wake of the attacks of September 11, 2001, and consider a sequence of particular events that have taken place over the twenty years that followed. The topics that I explore here are ones that I have been thinking about over the course of these two decades—through my doctoral studies in Science, Technology, and Society that I began in September 2001, through writing a dissertation about race and heart disease, and through more than a decade of teaching undergraduates about the intersections of biomedicine and culture and of science, technology, and race. Science, technology, and medicine both shape and are shaped by society and culture, and the racism that is pervasive both in health care settings and in broader society has consequences on both society and health. Each of the cases that I recount is *sickening* in at least two ways: provoking outrage and disgust and revealing multifaceted ways in which living in a racist society makes people sick.

The chapters take on diverse, familiar spheres of recognized urgency: terrorism, natural disaster, mass incarceration, police brutality, environmental justice, and reproductive justice. Each chapter is grounded in close attention to a concrete event that provides a distinctive window into those larger phenomena: the deaths of two Black postal workers in the 2001 anthrax attacks; the spike in chronic disease after Hurricane Katrina in 2005; the Scott sisters' case of 2010, in which double life sentences were suspended on condition of kidney donation; the preferential protection of General Motors machines rather than people at a key moment in the Flint water crisis in 2014; a teenage girl subjected to excessive force by a police officer at a 2015 suburban pool party; the life-threatening experience of childbirth for tennis star Serena Williams in 2017. *Sickening* shows that exceptional events can reveal the fundamental racialization of citizenship and health in the United States.

Each of the cases engages with health in different ways. Sometimes I write directly about medical care contexts, in which denial of care causes direct bodily harm and even death. But I also consider broader public spheres, not narrowly medical, as spaces that foster or inhibit bodily flourishing. Here, considering the World Health Organization definition of health is instructive: "health is a state of complete physical, mental and social well-being and not merely the absence of disease or infirmity."[3] Health is a capacious category, inextricable from the entire social world.

The six cases that I explore are a small portion of the egregious occurrences of the first two decades of the twenty-first-century United States. Although these cases are by no means comprehensive, there is a logic to their selection. Each offers opportunities to explore particular themes, and, taken together, they provide a more robust look into how racism harms health and well-being. Many additional topics could be covered, for example, anti-Black racism has structured the HIV/AIDS epidemic in the United States,[4] a vital public health issue that deserves sustained attention but does not find it here. I hope that readers will be informed by the six examples that are analyzed in this book as they grapple with other events—whether past events or events yet to come.

Attending to such wide-ranging examples foregrounds the multifaceted ways in which living in a structurally unequal society impacts the health and citizenship of racialized populations, especially African Americans. Racial disparities in medicine and health do not have a single cause but are the result of wide-ranging and interconnected elements of living in a racist society. In addition to the major themes of each of the particular chapters, *Sickening* draws attention throughout to structures that mediate health inequalities, ranging from encounters with health care providers to encounters with governmental authorities, in contexts of unequal infrastructures.

On one level, this book is a resource that I have wanted for use in my own undergraduate classroom. I strive to lay out the case studies and define key terms as I go, so that the chapters can be accessible to students with little background knowledge of the events and theories being discussed. Also, I have chosen topics and analytical frames with the goal of giving students a foundation in understanding key topics in racism and health. At the same time, no matter what level of background readers bring with them, I hope that this book is an opening to further engagement. To that end, I often identify and quote many scholars from diverse fields in the main text, rather than relegating that material exclusively to the footnotes, to characterize and invite readers into ongoing academic conversations of potential interest: there is much more worth reading. At the end of the book, I provide a set of analytical strategies that can be used as an assignment in an undergraduate classroom.

On another level, the book is also an interdisciplinary text that seeks to draw together and contribute to plural fields of scholarship, and I hope that graduate students and my colleagues in the social sciences and humanities will find its analysis rich enough to provide new insight. Readers who are unfamiliar with the scholarly debates might skim some sections within the chapters that attend to theoretical matters without worrying too much about the nuances, or they might become curious about them and follow the footnotes to explore them in more depth.

My focus is on the United States in particular, rather than taking a more global view, because attending to the specific national context is vital for understanding the historical and social constitution of racial inequality. At the same time, I strive to provide enough context and explanation that readers in many countries will find the accounts accessible and will be able to both appreciate the specificities and make transnational connections of their own.[5]

The selection of the twenty-first century is intentional, even as it will become clear that much longer histories matter tremendously. Many books about racism in medicine and health focus either on centuries-long histories starting with colonialism and slavery[6] or on famous twentieth-century cases that happened long before today's college students, and indeed many Americans, were even born, such as the Tuskegee Syphilis Study and the creation of the HeLa cell line from the cells of Henrietta Lacks.[7] As important as this history and these cases are, I have found in my teaching that reliance on them as the starting point for conversation can create an impression that the drivers of racial inequality in health are located in the past. This mode of narration sets up racism as a residual legacy of the past and, in so doing, elides the agency and responsibility of present-day actors and structures. By focusing specifically on twenty-first-century events, and following relevant historical threads without assuming either progress or stasis, this volume illuminates the ways in which these inequalities are constantly re-created in the present.

I start my account with an event that happened in 2001: the deaths of two Black postal workers in the anthrax attacks. The anthrax attacks have largely faded from public memory, in part because they happened just weeks after the large-scale terrorist attacks of September 11, 2001, and yet they are a useful starting point for this book. The September 11 attacks were more than just a large-scale tragic loss of life: they were truly extraordinary, the attacks themselves a spectacle. As I will discuss in the first chapter, the impact of those attacks was unusually democratic, in that people from all walks of life died as the planes crashed and the buildings collapsed. In the mass mourning of that time, there was a widespread media narrative that Americans, denizens of the most powerful country on earth, were now newly vulnerable. This obscured a more fundamental truth: that many Americans were never safe, and vulnerability has always been highly structured by race, gender, and class. After September 11, as before, Americans have never really been "all in this together," and attending to the deaths of the postal workers that occurred the following month helps to make that clear. The events that I analyze in this book are less spectacular than those of September 11, and the unequal impact that they have is far more ordinary. Although there is an element of spectacle in the events that I recount—they are, after all, events that garnered considerable attention—the unequal exposure to risk and the unjust denial of care are also profoundly routine. They are emblematic of the "slow violence" that often goes unnoticed but is fundamental to how bodily well-being becomes unequal.[8]

Another motivation for this starting point is worth highlighting. I specifically avoid starting my account where many other accounts of race and biomedicine in the twenty-first century begin—with an invocation of a ceremony on the White House lawn in 2000, at which President Bill Clinton announced that with the completion of the Human Genome Project, "one of the great truths to emerge from this triumphant expedition inside the human genome is that in genetic terms, all human beings, regardless of race, are more than 99.9 percent the same."[9] That is because, if we want to understand race and biomedicine today, the Human Genome Project is a poor jumping-off point. First, it implies that genetics is somehow fundamental to medicine and health, whereas genetics actually plays a relatively small role in medical care broadly, and a vanishingly small role in contributing to disparities in health outcomes.[10] Second, it puts the focus on the ontology of race—what race *is*—rather than foregrounding the far more important question of the impact of racism.[11]

ANTI-BLACK RACISM AND HEALTH DISPARITIES

From the book's subtitle, readers will notice that my focus is less on *race* and more on *racism*. Because of this focus on racism as a social practice,

I am not particularly interested in the problem of how racial categories are defined. Whereas many accounts of racism in science and technology studies focus on the *ambiguity* of race, I am more interested in its *durability*: the resilience of race as a concept in the face of constant critique and the amenability of racial disparities to provide not only an explanation of difference but a ground from which to demand change.[12] The enduring philosophical question of "who counts as Black?" is not one that is salient in any of the cases that I examine. On one level, this is because self-identified race has a very high correlation with socially defined race, especially for Americans who are white or Black. Even more fundamentally, when it comes to our health, how others define our race can have a greater impact on our health than how we define ourselves.[13]

The ways that race shapes experiences of health and medicine have far more to do with how others perceive us in snap judgments than with how we perceive ourselves in all our complexity. Racism operates in such a way that what matters most is whether authorities, ranging from physicians and police to teachers and mortgage officers, consider someone to be Black, not whether that Blackness might in some way be partial or contestable. This point is informed by historian Barbara Fields, who, writing about a 1999 case in which a Guinean immigrant named Amadou Diallo was shot by New York City police officers forty-one times in his own entryway while holding up his wallet, states,

> Diallo probably defined himself as a member of his nation or tribe or lineage, rather than as "black." But, under the American system, it was the officers' definition of him, not his definition of himself, that held the balance between life and death.[14]

Racial identities are not essences, then, but products of social processes. In keeping with the convention in much antiracist scholarship, I capitalize the term *Black* to highlight that it is a proper noun—a historically constituted social group rather than a physical description—and use the terms *African American* and *Black* interchangeably.[15] I am less interested in precisely naming and demarcating the categories than in attending to the unequal structuring of bodily experiences in a racist society.[16] In the

United States, increasing interest in gene frequencies, on one hand, and self-reported identity, on the other, has not displaced the reliance on a very particular commonsense visual convention in determining who counts as Black. As historian Evelynn Hammonds argues, "in the US race has always been dependent on the visual," and ideas about the mixing of what are conceived of as pure types does not displace this racial typology but reinforces it.[17] Any troubling of the categories does not undermine the impact of racism.

Racism impacts health in many ways. One helpful delineation comes from influential physician and epidemiologist Camara Jones, who outlines three "levels of racism":[18]

> *institutionalized racism*: "differential access to the goods, services, and opportunities in society by race," which "need not have an identifiable perpetrator" and "is often evident as inaction in the face of need."

> *personally mediated racism*: "prejudice and discrimination, where prejudice means differential assumptions about the abilities, motives, and intentions of others according to their race, and discrimination means differential actions toward others because of their race," and might be intentional or unintentional.

> *internalized racism*: "acceptance by members of the stigmatized races of negative messages about their own abilities and intrinsic worth."

Like Jones, I am most interested in the level of *institutionalized racism*, which is evident in differential exposures to harms (such as pollution) and differential access to assistance (such as medical care). *Personally mediated racism* is also often relevant, as enacted by people in positions of authority, ranging from police to health care providers. *Internalized racism* is largely beyond my scope, although there are occasional glimpses of it in quotes from key actors in the stories, and readers might reflect on how these events might produce such effects. All of these levels of racism contribute to *health disparities*, which is to say, the unequal burden of illness and unequal risk of death among different groups in society.

In broadly similar ways, many public health scholars have already characterized some of the same larger structural forces that my account seeks to illustrate. For example, Zinzi Bailey and colleagues describe "pathways between racism and health" in the medical journal *The Lancet,* including "economic injustice and social deprivation," "environmental and occupational health inequities," "psychosocial trauma," "inadequate healthcare," and several more elements.[19] The more intimate scale of the stories that I describe is meant to complement rather than replace this important work. The case study approach can help to bridge the conceptual gap between the important macrocosmic and quantitative research of epidemiologists and the microcosmic level of individual lives.

Although the topic of "racism and health disparities" should and could encompass attention to the structural issues and experiences of many groups of people in the United States, this book focuses on the effects of anti-Black racism on Black people in particular. Anti-Black racism plays a particularly pervasive role in the United States, and the cases in this book reveal diverse aspects of this singular topic. This is not to deny the impact of racism on other groups. Notably, racism fundamentally structures experiences of Native Americans, and of migrants from Latin America and their descendants, who are racialized in contested ways. Ideas about the inevitability of Indigenous illness have been foundational to notions of America as a settler colony,[20] and attending to the ways that those ideas are constantly renewed in the present demands a book of its own. The racialization of migrants from Latin America is intertwined with anti-Indigenous racism, while also emerging from particular borderland histories and xenophobic exacerbations in the present.[21] Indeed, poor and working-class white people's health is also negatively impacted by racism, because many white Americans would rather equal benefits be denied to others than support policies that would improve health and health care access for all.[22] Attention to the experiences of all these groups is an urgent and growing scholarship in its own right.

Some readers might question the focal framing of racism—surely some of the events described are fundamentally related to socioeconomic class inequality? Indeed, class matters a great deal, as will become clear in the chapters. Yet race cannot simply be displaced to class. In the United States, race and class are inextricably linked, and a desire to treat them as isolated variables is a desire to replace lived experience in the United States with an abstraction.[23] Experiences of race and class—as well as gender, sexuality, ability, and other stratifications of power—are not additive but intersectional.[24] Moreover, diverse phenomena ranging from segregated neighborhoods to disproportionately negative encounters with police and medical providers contribute to what public health scholar Nancy Krieger has characterized as the "accumulated insults" of living in a structurally racist society—facing repeated experiences with discrimination that takes forms that are indirect, direct (focused at individual-level discrimination), and population level (such as segregation).[25] No one individual's intersecting experiences can be completely separated from the individual's experiences as a member of a group. There might be places and times in which class identity fundamentally supersedes racial identity, but in the United States, fidelity to lived experience of inequalities demands a central focus on racism.

BIOPOLITICS AND CITIZENSHIP

Although the term *biopolitics* can be jargony—and certainly a great deal of scholarly ink has been spilled on its elaboration—it remains a useful idea. It is most associated with the late twentieth-century French theorist Michel Foucault. His discussion of the emergence of "biopower" in the modern age is instructive: "one might say that the ancient right to take life or let live was replaced by a power to *foster* life or *disallow* it to the point of death."[26] Foucault is highlighting a key contemporary aspect of the matter of the management of life: modern institutional power is not located so much in killing, as it was for premodern rulers, as it is in the differential between fostering (some) life and letting (others) die. Surveillance becomes a more pervasive mode of control than overt violence. The differential fostering of life operates in a way that is generally not spectacular but completely ordinary and routine.

There is a rich scholarship in the Foucauldian biopolitical tradition that attends to race, racism, and health. Sociologist Janet Shim's approach is perhaps most resonant with my own: she argues that race (and gender and class) should be reconceptualized as "social relations of power that are located not just in the biological bodies of individuals but in the social spaces between them, producing and stratifying the distribution of health and illness."[27] A larger share of this literature attends to the stakes of biomedical innovations, and this can sometimes be rather removed from the question of making live and letting die—focusing instead on the novel subjectivities produced as individuals come to understand themselves as biological subjects and seek to understand their history and optimize their health in the context of market-driven biomedicine.[28] These processes can become relevant for making live and letting die, for example, when biomedical ideas obscure rather than illuminate structural inequality. As sociologist Anthony Ryan Hatch argues in his analysis of the metabolic syndrome, this can be "the kind of biopolitics that simultaneously manufactures health problems and their remedies, deploys race as a way of concealing inequality," and constructs biomedical ideas precisely "to sever the relationship between body and society."[29] Moreover, some of the technology-oriented scholarship in the Foucauldian tradition provides insight into the question of differentially fostering life, especially of race-based pharmaceuticals and medical hot-spotting.[30] Even when these technologies promise to repair health disparities, they often instead increase surveillance of racialized populations without actually benefiting them. Sociocultural theorist Nadine Ehlers and geographer Shiloh Krupar provide a lucid introduction to Foucauldian biopower as they lay out their evocative concept of "deadly life-making," in which, in a racist society, the operations of forms of "making live" increase disparities and can even kill.[31]

The biopolitical sphere as we find it in this book is generally in the domain of ordinary life and routine medicine rather than novel sensibilities or genomic innovations. Distinctions between those whose lives are fostered and those whose lives are disregarded are constantly remade. For example, the differential availability of routine pharmaceuticals for acute and chronic diseases will be explored in the chapter on the deaths of the postal workers in the anthrax attacks and in the chapter on the increase in deaths from heart disease and diabetes after Hurricane Katrina. The differential exposure to harms, including carceral and environmental harms, will be explored in the chapters on the Scott sisters' case and the Flint water crisis, respectively. Various forms of surveillance remain central—now including state and medical surveillance as well as social media. One of the things that the biopolitical approach helps to highlight is that citizenship is about more than participation in electoral processes, and people's bodies as well as their political identities are at stake. Several chapters will touch on the plural senses of "biological citizenship" that emerge.

There is also a more fundamental notion of citizenship that inspires me, largely distinct from the Foucauldian tradition, that I want to bring to bear on this biopolitics. It comes from African American studies, notably political scientist Melissa Harris-Perry:

> If you ask most people what they think of when they hear the word *politics*, they are likely to give a definition that includes voters, parties, elections, public policy, and processes of contestation and representation. But formal participation in government is only one part of a more encompassing effort to be recognized within the nation. The struggle for recognition is the nexus of human identity and national identity, where much of the most important political work occurs.[32]

Contestation over citizenship in plural forms—some directly related to health and well-being, some indirectly related—emerges as a key theme of this book.

On one level, this theme of "citizenship" is a way to engage with who counts as an American citizen. There is a relatively narrow technical sense in which this matters: who is entitled and able to make demands on the U.S. government for services and care. There is also a broader, more representational sense in which it matters: who is discursively characterized as an authentic American and who is characterized as diversely outside the American public—as criminal, interloper, refugee in the aftermath of Hurricane Katrina—or as dependent in the carceral context of the Scott sisters, or as somehow less than fully human in the combination of hypervisibility and dehumanization of Serena Williams. In addition, I will engage with plural theoretical ideas of citizenship, ranging from "biological citizenship" to "corporate personhood." Sometimes citizenship struggles play out at an individual level: an individual person demanding rights and/or recognition. More often, however, citizenship struggles are mobilized by and for groups that, to at least some extent, precede any particular recognition demand. Consider Black Lives Matter: although that movement frames Blackness in somewhat different ways from the way that previous movements such as the civil rights movement have, it is building on that already existing political identity and making a recognition claim. Claiming to matter is claiming citizenship.[33]

NOTES ON METHOD AND APPROACH

My own training is in the interdisciplinary field of science, technology, and society (STS)—also called science and technology studies—and I am particularly attentive to a few key preoccupations of that interdisciplinary field. The first overlaps with a key Foucauldian idea: knowledge and power are inseparable. Epistemological concerns—that is, questions about how we come to know things—are inextricable from power. Although STS canonically tracks how scientific truth claims are made in laboratories,[34] this core insight is also relevant to understanding the wider world. The way that the credibility of truth claims is influenced by the social location of the speaker is illustrated many times over in this book when Black patients' complaints are not believed or taken seriously by their health care providers. As a second example, my attention is centrally on how the social and material inequalities that I track work *in practice*.[35] There is an emergent quality to structural racism and health inequalities that are not outside the social sphere in which they operate but constitute it. The third example is interest in both matter and meaning. The material and semiotic aspects of the events that I describe—their ability to shape both our bodies and our understanding—are inseparable, and both aspects are important.

Most scholarship in STS that focuses on the present is social scientific, employing qualitative research methods, such as interviews and participant observation, but this book is predominantly humanistic. This is not unique, and feminists who engage STS have been visionary in this kind of disciplinary boundary crossing—notably the foundational feminist STS theorist Donna Haraway[36] and a rich and growing body of Black feminist technoscience scholarship.[37] Feminists writing in sports studies have also articulated a resonant approach.[38] Although I hope to be in conversation with scholarship in the qualitative social sciences, especially anthropology and sociology, I take an interdisciplinary interpretive cultural studies approach: performing close readings of public events.[39] As Moya Bailey and Whitney Peoples have argued in their important call for a Black feminist health science studies, "media and health are co-constitutive," and media representations are an appropriate object for feminist technoscience analysis.[40]

Sickening attends closely to journalistic and academic accounts of each case to retell the stories of the specific events while putting them into a broader frame. If the stories were taken out of historical and social context and presumed to be able to operate analytically on their own, they would not provide persuasive analytical tools—the cases might be dismissed as anomalies. Putting the events into historical and contemporary social context helps to show the ways in which they reveal medicine as usual.

The stories that I have chosen are already publicly available and widely disseminated as cultural narratives. Thus I have purposely forgone interviews as a method. New interviews would not necessarily be more robust in terms of epistemic validity than the publicly available accounts and would have the potential of adding to the harm. Although I have certainly found interviewing to be useful in many projects, I am leery of performing my own interviews as a basis on which to ground stories of suffering. Asking people to retell their stories to me might authenticate my standing as a researcher, but it does not necessarily serve them. Feminist science and technology studies scholar Nassim Parvin's argument with regard to digital archiving projects is also relevant here: in our contemporary era, we are surrounded with such stories, which are all too often turned into commodities.[41] This is not to diminish the value of qualitative social science research, including into suffering, but to suggest that interviews might best be reserved for illuminating perspectives that are not already available as public narratives.[42] In my cases, I will leave the investigative journalism to the journalists and draw on already existing accounts to write a more interpretive account of my own.

My perspective is informed not only by my disciplinary training but also by my situatedness and experiences as an activist and an educator. Although I moved to London in 2018, I was born in the United States and lived there almost all my life. I was raised in rural northern Michigan, and I moved to cities on the East Coast and in the South for education and work: a couple of years each in Baltimore and Houston, a decade each in Boston and Atlanta. I spent ten years on the faculty at Georgia Tech, teaching such classes as Biomedicine and Culture and Science, Technology, and Race, and engaging with undergraduate students has been formative for my thinking. My hope is that this book provides useful teaching material for undergraduate students in the United States and beyond. Experiences beyond the academy have also been formative. I am a white lesbian who has been involved in activism for decades—especially feminist, queer, antiracist, and antiwar—and many of my commitments are rooted both in feminist and antiracist scholarship and in intersectional activism. Thus I have learned not only from my academic training but also from deep and long-standing engagement with students and with social justice advocates. My point of view is shaped by and accountable to distinct but overlapping academic and activist communities.

OVERVIEW OF THE BOOK

The chapters are written in such a way that they can be read individually, though reading them in combination is likely to be a richer experience. Reading multiple cases provides an opportunity to engage crosscutting themes across diverse examples and to explore the ways that structures that mediate health inequalities interlock and combine. The most accessible chapters are chapter 1 and chapter 6. The middle chapters are a bit more challenging because they delve into complicated concepts: biopolitics (chapter 2), biological citizenship (chapter 3), more than human politics (chapter 4), and race as technology (chapter 5).

Chapter 1 examines the case of two Black postal workers, Thomas

Morris and Joseph Curseen, who died of inhalation anthrax on October 21, 2001. These postal workers' deaths took place in a defining moment in U.S. history, making the case a fitting one with which to open this book focused on racism and health in the twenty-first century. The chapter is anchored especially by the transcript of a telephone call to the emergency number 911 that one of the postal workers made hours before he died, recounting his unsuccessful pursuit of treatment for what he had rightly suspected was anthrax. Returning to this event provides a fresh perspective into the continuities and discontinuities at the dawn of the twenty-first century. Although the postal workers' deaths were extraordinary, their experiences provide a valuable focal point for thinking about political and medical systems that routinely fail to provide adequate care to African Americans. In this chapter, I focus on three intertwined elements: the justifiable suspicion among African Americans that neither the state nor the medical system prioritizes their care; the reluctance to recognize Black suffering among officials, physicians, and mainstream media; and how this event—which happened so soon after September 11, 2001—already revealed as a lie the then-powerful narrative that in the post–September 11 world, Americans were "all in this together."

In chapter 2, I discuss the unnatural disaster of chronic disease after Hurricane Katrina. Hurricane Katrina hit southeast Louisiana in late August 2005. The levees that protected New Orleans failed; 80 percent of the city was flooded—mostly residential areas—and thousands died. In the initial days after the storm, public health experts worried about the spread of infectious disease. However, chronic diseases, such as cardiovascular disease and diabetes, emerged as the far greater threat. In this chapter, I attend to the ways in which lack of access to care contributed to increased chronic disease, focusing especially on one particular, tangible element: pharmaceuticals. I track the travels of pharmaceuticals in the aftermath of Hurricane Katrina to explore three key ways in which the response to the emergency exacerbated the preexisting vulnerability of the population, especially with regard to health: at emergency shelters, in drug donation programs, and in ongoing care. Each of these disrupted pharmaceutical flows provides an opportunity to see ways that those most acutely impacted by Hurricane Katrina were framed as outside of the "mainstream

American public," in intertwining ways. Disrupted pharmaceutical flows at emergency shelters exemplify the ways in which Katrina victims were impacted by discourses and practices associated with criminality; disrupted pharmaceutical flows in drug donation programs do the same with regard to subjects of global health charity; disrupted pharmaceutical flows in ongoing care illuminate their marginalization. Being outside ordinary pharmaceutical flows and being outside the "American public" occur through mutually reinforcing processes. The chapter concludes with discussion of biopolitics, as elaborated in Foucault's important lecture "Society Must Be Defended," to argue that being ideologically defined as outside of society has material consequences for racist distributions of mortality.

Chapter 3 explores the impact of mass incarceration through attention to the case of the Scott sisters. In December 2010, the governor of Mississippi suspended the dual life sentences of two African American sisters who had been imprisoned for sixteen years on an extraordinary condition: that Gladys Scott donate a kidney to her ailing sister Jamie Scott. The Scott sisters' case is a highly unusual one, yet it is a revealing site for inquiry into U.S. biopolitics more broadly. Close attention to the conditional release and its context demands a broader frame than traditional bioethics. This chapter draws on the Scott sisters' case as a site for interrogating the U.S. context of racialized mass incarceration. Tensions between racialized exclusions, the promise of consumerist freedom, and their lack of expectations of the state are foundational to a distinctly American biological citizenship. By putting the Scott sisters' case into conversation with broader arguments about incarceration as a site of racialization and anthropological literatures of organ transplantation and of biological citizenship in diverse geographical sites, this chapter seeks to articulate some of the racialized contours of biopolitics in the United States.

In the fourth chapter, I attend to one small element of the Flint water crisis: the swift provision of clean water to the General Motors engine plant even as the people of Flint were abandoned for years. In April 2014, the city of Flint, Michigan, began drawing on a new source of water as part of fiscal austerity measures. Almost immediately, Flint's human residents complained about the look and smell of the new water, but these complaints were dismissed and ignored by city managers for years. Representatives of the most prominent nonhuman corporate resident of Flint—General Motors (GM)—complained about the water quickly, too, because the new water supply was corroding the machinery at their Flint engine plant. But only GM was able to change water sources before the damage to the pipes became permanent. The chapter follows such disparate nonhuman objects as fiscal bonds, machines, and pipes to track the intertwined flows of capital, labor, and water. In this chapter, I argue that the differential protection of the nonhuman material integrity of GM's machines over the nonhuman material integrity of the water pipes and the human bodily integrity of the people of Flint provides a window into racialized biopolitics. The protection of finance and machines over infrastructure and people illustrates the devaluation of groups of humans considered to be surplus in the service of the interests of capital. It also demonstrates the extent to which ideas of emergency, citizenship, and bodily integrity are politically contingent. This small event within the broader Flint water crisis illustrates a fundamental element of racial disparities in health in the United States: differential protection of nonhuman financial capital and racialized human life.

Chapter 5 analyzes an infamous instance of police brutality at a pool party. In June 2015, fifteen-year-old Dajerria Becton was among the African American teenagers at a pool party in the Dallas suburb of McKinney, Texas, who were violently suppressed by the police. The incident was captured on cell phone videos that were widely disseminated, which included a powerful image of the small bikini-clad girl's bodily vulnerability under the knee of a police officer. Close attention to the McKinney case reveals ways in which racism and antiracism are renewed and refigured in the twenty-first century. In this chapter, I articulate and put into relation the plural technologies of race (and gender) that came together in this encounter and its aftermath: suburban communities and swimming pools, bikinis and police uniforms, cell phone cameras and social media. This chapter explores the spatial and social relations specific to a homeowners association–managed community pool and puts that into relationship with the role of the police in enforcing segregation. The chapter also foregrounds the role of social media in distributing focal images for righteous anger, while arguing for the value of deeper engagement with the incidents and their contexts to more fully explicate what they reveal about unjust social structures. It engages the literature of "race as technology" and the "liberatory imagination" to explore how artists and activists are mobilizing images as part of advocacy for justice.

In chapter 6, I explore tennis star Serena Williams's life-threatening experience when giving birth to her daughter in September 2017 as a window into reproductive injustice. That someone with so much wealth, power, and expertise faced such challenges receiving the care that she needed exposes the inadequacy of frequently invoked explanations for high maternal mortality among Black women, such as poverty or failure to seek prenatal care. The chapter then puts Williams's account of her experience into the context of two intersecting elements: links between her birth experience and those of far too many Black women, and representations of her body over the course of her career to illuminate the ways in which Black women's bodies are simultaneously hypersurveilled and inadequately cared for. Williams is not an uncomplicated figure in this landscape, but when she mobilizes her social media platform to call attention to racially stratified access to safe births and to demand change, she contributes to reproductive justice advocacy.

The book's conclusion explores some of the ways that the cases analyzed in this book provide insight into the twinned events of summer 2020: the crisis of COVID-19 and the resurgence of Black Lives Matter. It draws together what has been learned by looking across domains—workplaces, communities, institutions, leisure spaces, infrastructures—underscoring the value of considering wholes and parts. It also provides a set of analytical strategies on which readers can draw to form analyses of other events, presented in a way that can be modified for use in wide-ranging classroom contexts: an iterative four-step template for analysis that I call the *sickening assignment*. Finally, it encourages readers to combine analysis and additional action.

1

Terrorism

THE DEATHS OF BLACK POSTAL WORKERS
IN THE 2001 ANTHRAX ATTACKS

OPERATOR: Hello.

MORRIS: Yes, um, my name is Thomas L. Morris Jr., I'm at 4244 Suitland
Road in the [mumble] apartment complex, apartment 201.

OPERATOR: And what's the problem?

MORRIS: My breathing is very, very labored.

OPERATOR: How old are you?

MORRIS: Um, fifty-five.

MORRIS: Ah, I, I don't know if I have been, but I suspect that I might have
been exposed to anthrax.[1]

Two Black postal workers, Thomas Morris and Joseph Curseen,
died of inhalation anthrax on October 21, 2001. Their deaths have largely
receded from public memory. Although this event was extraordinary,
attending to it provides a valuable focal point for consideration of political and medical systems that routinely fail to provide adequate care to
African Americans.[2]

These postal workers' deaths took place in a defining moment in
U.S. history, making the case a fitting one with which to open this book
focused on racism and health in the twenty-first century. In both academic
and broader public discussions of African American distrust of medical
providers, it is conventional to hearken back to the infamous Tuskegee
Syphilis Study of 1932–72, a U.S. Public Health Service study of the natural
course of untreated syphilis that continued long after treatment that could
have cured the men was discovered.[3] Yet even as Tuskegee stands as a
landmark breach of clinical research ethics, we need not look so far back

to find poignant examples of denial of life-saving medical care. Indeed, although references to Tuskegee were a recurring theme in focus groups held with Black postal workers in D.C. after the anthrax attacks,[4] distrust is not a lingering legacy but a constantly re-created present. Although my focus in this chapter is on health care in a crisis rather than on clinical research, my account is aligned with the important intervention from sociologist Ruha Benjamin about the roots of African American distrust of medical research: Benjamin "challenges the conventional focus on 'African-American distrust' as a set of attitudes grounded in collective memories of past abuses and projected on to current initiatives, by examining the sociality of distrust produced daily in the clinic and reinforced in broader politics of health investment."[5]

In this chapter, I focus on three intertwined elements: the justifiable suspicion among African Americans that neither the state nor the medical system prioritizes their care; the reluctance to recognize Black suffering among officials, physicians, and mainstream media; and how this event—which happened so soon after September 11, 2001—already revealed as a lie the then-powerful narrative that in the post–September 11 world, Americans were "all in this together."

In October 2001, four letters containing anthrax were mailed by an unknown perpetrator: two were mailed to journalists, and two were mailed to senators. The anthrax-containing letter sent to Senator Tom Daschle was processed at the Brentwood Postal Facility in Northeast Washington, D.C., on October 11, 2001. When it was opened by an intern four days later, on October 15, the Capitol building was immediately evacuated, and all who worked there were given the broad-spectrum antibiotic drug Cipro as a precaution and then were subject to testing before continuing on the longer course of the antibiotic if necessary. The entire Capitol building was thoroughly cleaned while evacuated.

Meanwhile, unknown to anyone at the time, anthrax contamination from that letter remained at the Brentwood Postal Facility, whose employees were told they were not at risk and should continue working.

The disease was incubating in at least four postal workers. One of them, Joseph Curseen, went to the emergency room on October 16 complaining of flu-like symptoms, suspecting the cause might have been food poisoning. He was treated for dehydration and nausea and sent away without being tested for anthrax. After collapsing on October 21, he returned to the hospital and died there the next day. Another postal worker, Thomas Morris, went to a primary care doctor on October 18 complaining of flu-like symptoms and informing the doctor that he believed he had been exposed to anthrax. His doctor took a swab but diagnosed it as a flu virus and sent Morris away with advice to take Tylenol for achiness. Morris was never informed of the results of that swab. Three days later, before dawn on October 21, still more ill, he made a call to 911 and was taken by ambulance to the hospital. He died there eleven hours later.

One of the infected workers who would survive, Leroy Richmond, sought treatment on October 19 for his flu-like symptoms first from the Brentwood facility nurse, who told him he had a low-grade fever but nothing to worry about. The doctor at his health maintenance organization center likewise told him that he did not seem very sick. Continuing on to the emergency room, his case was not initially seen as major, but he insisted on staying. When the attending physician came on duty, she immediately began treating him for anthrax pending outcome of his tests. Richmond's daughter acted as his advocate throughout the four-week treatment, double-checking his care with a physician she knew personally. The treatment was successful, and Richmond was released from the hospital on November 13.[6]

As of this writing in 2020, there is still no definitive answer as to who perpetrated the attacks. Writing five years after the attacks in 2006, Senator Daschle himself lamented that the investigation's trail had "gone cold" and that the public health infrastructure remained inadequate to the task of dealing with future attacks.[7] Among postal workers reflecting on that five-year anniversary, desires for forgiveness and healing remained intertwined with bitterness and a sense of ongoing vulnerability.[8] The case shows no sign of closing.

But let's return to October 2001.

MORRIS: But I am—my breathing is labored and my chest feels constricted. Um, I am getting air, but to get up and walk and what have you, I feel like I might just pass out and stuff if I stand up too long, so I'm just chillin'.

OPERATOR: OK, which post office do you work at?

MORRIS: This is the post office downtown, um, Brentwood Road, Washington, D.C., post office. [pause] There was, ah, a woman found an envelope, and I was in the vicinity. It had powder in it. They never let us know whether the thing had anthrax or not. They never, ah, treated the people who were around this particular individual and the supervisor who handled the envelope. Ah, so I don't know if it is or not. I'm just, I haven't been able to find out, I've been calling. But the symptoms that I've had are what was described to me in a letter they put out, almost to a tee. Except I haven't had any vomiting, except just until a few minutes ago. I'm not bleeding, and I don't have diarrhea. The doctor thought that it was just a virus or something, so we went with that and I was taking Tylenol for the achiness. Except the shortness of breath now, I don't know, that's consistent with the, with the anthrax.

OPERATOR: OK, you weren't the one that handled the envelope, it was somebody else?

MORRIS: No, I didn't handle it, but I was in the vicinity.

OPERATOR: OK, and do you know what they did with the envelope?

MORRIS: I don't know anything. I don't know anything. I couldn't even find out if the stuff was or wasn't. I was told that it wasn't, but I have a tendency not to believe these people.

Most media attention to these men's deaths at the time was focused on the poignant disparity of treatment on a macrocosmic level: while anthrax's threat to congressional workers was if anything overaddressed, the threat to postal workers was denied without investigation until men died. At Capitol Hill, even the dogs were tested and treated,[9] while at the Brentwood Postal Facility, officials went on the assessment of the Centers for Disease Control and Prevention (CDC) that postal workers were safe.[10] As the *Baltimore Sun* put it after the postal workers' deaths, "postal employees angrily questioned why they had been working in an anthrax hot zone when Capitol Hill was in the process of shutting down. Some wondered whether decisions favored the powerful: well-heeled congressional staff were tested but working-class mail carriers were not."[11]

At the Capitol, officials erred on the side of caution, whereas postal workers were repeatedly told that there was nothing to worry about. Although it was not a single actor who made the decision to close the Capitol but not the post office—the former decision was made by the attending physician of the U.S. Capitol, while the latter decision was made by the U.S. Postal Service in consultation with the CDC—from the perspective of people at risk, such a highly visible contrast was galling.[12] Several postal workers pointed out the contradiction, among them Vanessa Slaughter: "With Congress, they shut them down, had them tested, didn't let them go back to work. But they didn't do anything for us. We should have been tested a long time ago. Instead they just said: 'Y'all will be all right.'"[13] U.S. homeland security advisor Tom Ridge answered the concern with unambiguously class-conscious language, saying that health officials "weren't looking at the collar of their shirts, whether it was a white-collar or a blue-collar challenge."[14]

While postal workers often do in fact wear blue shirts as part of their uniforms, the focus on class in the mainstream press coverage reveals only part of the story. Ignored in that coverage is both the racial character of the Postal Service and the relative class *privilege* these men had vis-à-vis much of the Black community, particularly of Washington, D.C. As Wiley Hall wrote in the *Washington Afro-American,* "it is a little ironic to find postal employees among the ranks of the little people. I am a native of Washington. I grew up at a time when postal employees ranked among the most respected members of the community, along with doctors, teachers, undertakers, and military officers. Postal employees had a steady income with generous benefits. They owned their homes. They sent their children to college. They served as deacons in the church."[15]

The Postal Service has long played an important role as an employment opportunity for African Americans. For decades, the Postal Service was the only federal employer that employed African Americans, and at the turn of the twenty-first century, it remained the largest civilian employer of African Americans.[16] Frances Beal of the Black Radical Congress was among those who underscored the particular racial character of the Postal Service, particularly in Washington, D.C., in observing the response to the anthrax attacks. Racism in the private sector has historically meant that many Blacks with master's and even doctoral degrees have turned to jobs at the Postal Service as a "fallback," and Beal writes that "many union members are convinced that the racial composition of the workers at risk plays a part in the casual attitude of the quasi-federal postal service toward the workers' health and safety."[17]

In the Black press at the time, several writers noted their own families' experiences in discussing the role that the post office has played in employing relatively privileged African Americans.[18] At ESPN.com, Ralph Wiley wrote to this point with poignant humor referencing the movie *Hollywood Shuffle,* in which Black actors who refuse stereotyped roles console themselves with the mantra "There's always work at the post office." Wiley draws a further connection to professional sports as he plays off that line:

> "There's always work at the Post Office." That was a line from the movie "Hollywood Shuffle." Yeah. *Dangerous* work.
>
> You can be a big enough, good enough athlete to make the NFL, be hospitalized with a chest contusion, collapsed lung, or bruised sternum, unable to draw breath without pain. Or you can learn the sorting scheme, work at the P.O., end up anthraxed, hospitalized, unable to draw breath without pain.

Wiley also underscores the connection these postal workers had with D.C.'s mayor, who was vociferously denying that any bias was involved in the response to anthrax:

> The mayor of Washington is a Wally Cox act-alike named Anthony Williams, as Ivy-educated, bow-tied, and accountancy as all-get-out. Both his parents worked their entire careers at the post office. Raised eight kids doing it.

And Wiley concludes with what he himself calls "old jokes, dead jokes, stale jokes":

> "What do you call the white man in a huddle with 10 black men? Quarterback."
>   "What do you call a white man ordering 10,000 black people carrying bags? Postmaster."[19]

The community so overrepresented in post offices across the country is especially overrepresented in Washington, D.C., with its particularly stark racial stratification. According to one estimate, 92 percent of the employees at the Brentwood Postal Facility at the time were Black.[20]

The class character of the workers at the Brentwood facility cannot be divorced from their race. Much of the literature about racial disparities in health care in the post–civil rights era focuses on poverty and lack of education[21] or failure among African Americans to seek care.[22] But these men were not in poverty, and, complete with health insurance, they did seek care. To the extent that they were working class, they were so also in its positive sense—employed and nonpoor, relatively well educated and well compensated compared with most African Americans. Curseen even owned his own home and was active in that quintessentially middle-class type of club, the homeowners association.[23] Both were natives of the District, and both had moved out to the middle-class Black community of Prince Georges County, Maryland. Curseen was a college graduate,[24] and Morris was well informed enough to be alert to the signs of anthrax. But that information was not enough.

> OPERATOR: And did you tell your doctor that this is what happened?
> MORRIS: Huh?
> OPERATOR: Did you tell the doctor?
> MORRIS: Yes, I did. But he said that he didn't think that it was that. He thought that it was probably a virus or something.
> OPERATOR: I'm going to get the call into the ambulance.
> *[long pause; Morris breathes laboriously]*

Given that the postal workers were not systematically given testing and treatment by their governmental employers, there remains another layer that I have not seen explored in the mainstream or scholarly media. Setting aside the fact that the state did not initiate testing and treatment for these men, why were their own efforts to seek it out also unsuccessful? The failures of medical health care at the level of the physicians these men sought out remains to be explored, and race is implicated in this failure as well.

Concern about misuse of antibiotics was, evidently, something officials and physicians considered particularly risky when it came to Black postal workers. Responding to criticism after Morris and Curseen died, Dr. Mitch Cohen of the CDC said, "There is a risk in prophylaxis when it is not necessary. One of our basic goals is to identify who is at risk. Previous investigations in Florida and New York did not identify that the postal workers were at risk." However, according to the same report, "On Capitol Hill, more that 3,000 people were readily given Cipro in the two days after Daschle's letter was opened. Some of the people lining up to get tested and receive the antibiotic said they had not been in the building where the anthrax spilled but simply wanted the medication for reassurance."[25] In the weeks that followed, the governmental medical system had given up any pretense of trying to prevent misuse of antibiotics and showered postal workers with the drugs without providing universal testing.[26] D.C.'s top health official, Ivan Walks, had clearly disregarded concern for conservative use of antibiotics when he said on October 23 that "We do not need to do further testing, but we do need to treat quickly."[27]

In that tumultuous fall of 2001, I was a PhD student at the Massachusetts Institute of Technology (MIT), and I personally knew several (white) worry warts who at the height of the general anxiety about anthrax had their doctors prescribe them a bit of Cipro "just in case," and the letters page of the *New York Times* included many such reports throughout October and November. As a middle-class white woman quite comfortable with and demanding of doctors (and who has even had Cipro prescribed to me in the past), I am sure that I could have acquired Cipro had I sought it out.[28] At a contemporaneous "Technology and Self" luncheon organized by MIT professor Sherry Turkle to discuss pharmacology and identity

(RxID) with a Pfizer middle manager, the speaker mentioned that "anyone in this room could get a prescription for Cipro if they wanted." (There were, as is common at events of this sort at MIT, no Black people in the room.) At the time of that talk, I didn't have the chance to ask, if these drugs are so easy for us to access, why couldn't these postal workers get the drugs they needed in time?

Here, there is a connection to racial profiling in health care, in particular as to whether African Americans are believed by physicians—both to be really sick and to be sufficiently treatment compliant. On one hand, African Americans are often stereotyped as "drug-seeking" and differentially denied medicines for pain, among other conditions.[29] On the other hand, health care providers are less likely to provide optimal treatment for African Americans on the basis of stereotypes that these patients will not be compliant anyway.[30] The anthrax attack postal worker survivor, Leroy Richmond, has told his story of surviving anthrax as one of having to fight to be believed by doctors.[31] Richmond credits his survival to his skepticism, and that quality does seem to be what set Richmond apart from his deceased coworkers (and friends). Curseen and Morris either could not or did not question their physicians.

> OPERATOR: Do you know when?
> MORRIS: It was last, what, last Saturday a week ago, last Saturday morning at work. I work for the Postal Service. I've been to the doctor. Ah, I went to the doctor Thursday, he took a culture, but he never got back to me with the results. I guess there was some hang-up over the weekend, I'm not sure. But in the meantime, I went through a achiness and headachiness. This started Tuesday. Now I'm having difficulty breathing, and just to move any distance, I feel like I'm going to pass out. I'm here at the house, my wife is here, I'm on the couch.

Some editorials have operated on the assumption that believing public officials is what led to the deaths of Curseen and Morris. For example, an angry editorial titled "So-Called Little People Get Left Out of Loop" in the *Buffalo News* read, "For the record, the two workers who believed [Postmaster General] Potter and [CDC director] Koplan were named

Joseph P. Curseen, Jr. and Thomas L. Morris Jr."[32] But in fact only Curseen seems to have believed what officials told him; Morris suspected his bosses were not being honest.

However, Morris's case shows that it is not enough to be skeptical of officials wherever they are in that chain of command—CDC, postmaster general, or postal supervisors—that decided that postal workers as a group did not need testing and treatment; a Black man seeking adequate health care needs also to be skeptical of his doctor. In his 911 call made on day 5 of his illness and just eleven hours before his death, Morris described his earlier attempts to seek treatment. As he explained to the 911 operator, Morris had believed he had been exposed to anthrax at his job, and he had told his doctor that when he sought out his care promptly upon becoming ill. However, rather than providing Morris with antibiotics pending the results of the test for anthrax, the doctor told Morris that he had the flu and sent him home with Tylenol.

In the 911 call, Morris expressed his skepticism toward his governmental employers, saying of a suspicious substance found shortly before he became ill, "I was told that it wasn't [anthrax], but I have a tendency not to believe these people."[33] However, he may have believed his doctor for far too long. "The doctor thought that it was just a virus or something, so we went with that, and I was taking Tylenol for the achiness." Morris sounds both more team oriented and more trusting when speaking about his relationship with his doctor than when speaking of his employers; Morris seems to have accepted the doctor's assessment of his condition as his own. Speaking on behalf of Morris's son, lawyer Jimmy Bell pointed out, "He informed his physician right up front that he believed that he was exposed to anthrax. He believed his doctor. You're not going to question your physician. When he tells you what it is, that's what it is."[34]

The doctor displayed considerable incompetence, failing to get the results of the swab. But Morris still seemed deferential to him, rather than angry: "I guess there was some hang-up over the weekend."[35]

The medical literature on the case omits the fact that Morris had informed his doctor of his suspicions of anthrax on his initial visit. An authorial team of several physicians, led by physicians affiliated with the Johns Hopkins Center for Civilian Biodefense Studies, published a paper in the *Journal of the American Medical Association* detailing the cases of Curseen and Morris, respectively:

> Both patients in this report sought medical care for apparently mild, nonspecific illnesses and were sent home. Only after the news media reported cases of inhalational anthrax involving 2 postal workers from the local mail facility did these patients' physicians consider the possibility that they could have inhalational anthrax. At that point, the patients had been ill for 7 days (patient 1) and 5 days (patient 2).[36]

In this rendering, the concerns of a sick patient are not something that affects the possibilities that a physician considers. And yet this dismissal is fundamental to why Morris in particular did not survive. What made Curseen and Morris vulnerable, then, was the dismissive attitude not only of the state but also of their doctors. Skepticism toward doctors is what differentiated the case of a survivor, Leroy Richmond. The *New York Times* never published a comprehensive article analyzing the cases of all the anthrax-affected postal workers, but it did profile Richmond, describing him as the one that "wouldn't take no for an answer":

> "When the doctor said, 'I hear a little wheezing, but it's nothing to be concerned about,' I'm thinking, 'Well, he's the doctor, but I just don't believe him,'" he said. . . .
>
> Mr. Richmond said he has since come to conclude that the difference between living and dying on those pivotal few days was whether or not you believed what you were told. The two men who died, Joseph P. Curseen Jr. and Thomas L. Morris Jr., both saw doctors and were sent home. Mr. Richmond simply would not leave.[37]

Crucially, Richmond also had an advocate, his daughter, Alicia Richmond Scott. Scott was a program analyst at the Department of Health and Human Services and had a physician friend frequently on the phone to give her advice about what critical levels of tests and measurements to "keep an eye on." She also constantly questioned the nurses and interns assigned to the intensive care unit for information about her father's case and "then used that information to go back and challenge the attending doctors."[38] Scott's proactive participation in the care of her father not only helped prevent his case from falling through the cracks but actually contributed to the design of the successful medical treatment. Skepticism about doctors' opinions and a strong and capable advocate, then, were both important elements of Richmond's ability to tell his story of survival.

Thomas Morris's son filed a $37 million suit against Kaiser Permanente alleging that the HMO's doctor failed to provide the standard of care and that Morris faced racial bias when sent home without antibiotics. The suit was settled a year later, and the physician involved will likely never go public with any explanation.[39] But we can speculate that Morris sounded perhaps as paranoid to his doctor as he did on his 911 call. How can a doctor tell a paranoid Black man who believes that the government is lying to him from a rational Black man who believes that the government is lying to him?

> MORRIS, *mumbling*: I'm trying to put my pants on. So what do I need for, just my, my health care is Kaiser. So just bring my card and my . . .
> OPERATOR: Yes. You're gonna need your . . . did the doctor give you any kind of medication or anything?
> MORRIS: No, he just told me to take Tylenol for the achiness.

Kaiser Permanente, having been the one sued by the Morris family, issued prompt denials that its physician acted inappropriately in failing to quickly assess test results and provide treatment in light of Morris's concerns. The HMO did not address Morris's statements to his doctor but only the statements made by the officials of the CDC and the Postal Service, arguing that Kaiser had "meticulously followed the guidance they had at the time."[40] Kaiser spokeswoman Susan Whyte Simon maintained that "what we did was proportionate to his symptoms and what we knew about anthrax and who was at risk at the time. We think we did the right things."[41]

Moreover, Kaiser officials emphasized the actions of the HMO with regard to all of the victims, rather than just the case of Morris. Again quoting spokesperson Simon:

We will defend their allegations quite vigorously and with great passion. We are proud of the care delivered by Kaiser Permanente physicians and the information that our medical staff has provided to advance medical knowledge in treating anthrax. Our physicians were in the vanguard of diagnosing and treating anthrax.[42]

Kaiser's claim to have delivered effective treatment for anthrax is not completely groundless—although it failed to treat those who died, other postal workers on its health plan fared better. Leroy Richmond, as we have seen, fought his way to adequate care and survived. One other victim, unnamed, was also insured by Kaiser and survived.[43] This line of argument is an interesting insight into the logic of managed care and its discontents. According to this logic, denial of adequate care to an individual is not something that can be considered independent of the care that others receive. The survival of Richmond and another anthrax victim can be used as evidence to deny that Morris received inadequate treatment. By Kaiser's logic, a 66 percent survival rate of anthrax and some success at minimizing unnecessary antibiotics prescriptions should be good enough.

Many have argued that the U.S.-specific health insurance paradigm known as "managed care" has its own moral logic that is distinct from that of medicine. According to medical anthropologist Tanya Luhrmann, in both biomedicine and psychotherapy, "the patient is an end in himself. The patient is the sole person, more or less, on whom the doctor's care is focused, and the moral compass of the doctor's attention settles directly on the patient and the patient's immediate environment."[44] Not complicating the matter with a recognition of the old paternalism's dual nature (both condescending and caring), Luhrmann argues that this dyad becomes a triad under managed care:

> When the doctor enters the managed care system, that is no longer the case. The patient's care is managed relative to the needs of the group of which the patient is a part. A third party intervenes between the doctor and the patient, and the doctor must convince that third party of the patient's needs.[45]

Although Luhrmann here seems to idealize the old-fashioned practice of medicine, which was never so pure and certainly has never really extended fully to African Americans, the change in the logic is still important: it changes the justification for maltreatment. The shifting paternalist dyad justified maltreatment of African Americans by not recognizing their full humanity—as when slaves were experimented upon and when Blacks were denied care at Tuskegee[46]—and by excluding them from care by segregation and economics. Thus, African Americans have never been full beneficiaries of the paternalist dyad. Yet the managed care triad is no less hazardous for this marginalized group.

In a model in which there is a limited good to be distributed, managed care operates by trying to minimize all medical treatments, including the number of prescriptions. Especially in a crisis, the decision of whom to treat is not based on the needs of individual patients. Since not all individuals can be feasibly tested and treated, a certain number of individuals will be systematically shortchanged by managed care. In a structurally racist society, those shortchanged individuals will disproportionately be Black.[47] The reversion to this default reinforces the long-standing confluence of the refusal to recognize Black suffering and the acquiescence to white patients' demands for time, treatment, and reassurance from medical practitioners.

Moreover, the shorter time spent by doctors with individual patients encourages use of snap judgments about who is likely to be telling the truth about their condition and who is likely to be treatment compliant. Those pressures are enacted through racial profiling in health care. At the time of these events in the fall semester of 2001, I was in a class on the social studies of biomedicine at Harvard Medical School, where Professor Evelynn Hammonds spoke about the need to resist racial profiling in health care. Several of the doctors-to-be took offense at her call. They insisted that they would always take a full medical history and that they would never assume based on race that a particular individual was likely to be misinformed or unmotivated to follow through with treatment. However, Hammonds called the class's attention to the fact that this issue is larger than individual doctors' attitudes: the "medical history" itself is part of the racialized practice of health care, with race appearing as a blank to fill in or a box to check right up top, and without continually heightened vigilance, these future physicians are unlikely to be able to break out of the common framework that uses that categorization to make a range of other judgments.

Asserting that they would have required absurdly specific knowledge to justify testing and treatment of postal workers, CDC director Koplan said simply, "We had had no cases of inhalation anthrax in a mail-sorting facility. There was no reason to think this was a possibility."[48] Except for common sense, perhaps not. Neither had they reason to believe that an entire building on Capitol Hill needed to be evacuated, nor that dogs needed to be tested and treated, nor that workers who had not been in the building at the time needed to be tested and treated. Nonetheless, they took these extensive measures. When it came to the Capitol, they erred on the side of caution. When it came to Black postal workers, they erred on the side of carelessness.

The CDC's expert knowledge about the spread of anthrax spores excluded obviously relevant local knowledges, such as that of postal workers:

> In his truck, Clarence Raynor usually listens to WTOP as he ferries mail from Brentwood to neighborhood post offices and back, and on the afternoon of Oct. 15, the all-news station told him that a letter that might have anthrax spores had arrived in the Hart offices of Senate Majority Leader Thomas A. Daschle (D-S.D.). Raynor, though a postal worker for only four years, knew the arteries of delivery in the city, and he knew that the Daschle letter must have passed through Brentwood. "If he's contaminated," Raynor thought, meaning Daschle, "we're contaminated."
>
> Not that Raynor, 48, is an expert in how bacteria can penetrate or float. But he knew what sorting machines do to a piece of mail. "It is shaken, bounced around, pulled at, tugged at, beat up. . . . It is not just sitting still." And he knew how the machines were cleaned, how dust and scraps were blown. "They do it with pressurized air. It's like an air hose at a service station."[49]

Had the CDC solicited the knowledge of postal workers, it would have been able to make better recommendations on testing and treatment.[50]

Newsday was characteristically blunt in response to official denials of responsibility: postal workers "do not want to hear from the president of the United States, the head of the Centers for Disease Control, the postmaster general, or the district's mayor or any other talking head with a wagging tongue, that everyone moved to protect them as quickly as they know how. Experience tells them this is laughable or a bald lie, take your pick."[51]

Here, we begin to see ruptures in "United We Stand." And officials responded predictably by wrapping themselves in the American flag. According to Postmaster General John E. "Jack" Potter, "this is not a situation where Americans should be pointing fingers at anyone else other than the terrorists." On a similar note, President Bush's spokesperson Ari Fleisher said of Curseen and Morris, "The president believes that the cause of death was not the treatment made by the federal government or the local officials, or anybody else, that the cause of death was the attack that was made on our nation as a result of people mailing anthrax through the mail."[52] Never mind that there is no evidence that the perpetrator of the anthrax attacks was foreign, or that it is hardly comforting that despite the terrorists' targeting of powerful white men (Daschle in this case), Black men were the ones who died.[53]

Addressing the question of whether more concern should have been given to the potential risk to those who were exposed to the anthrax-containing letter before it was opened, Surgeon General David Satcher, in hindsight, said there should have been; he was the only official who said in so many words "we were wrong."[54] Satcher's job was mostly a symbolic one, and he lacked any executive power over the case,[55] but as one of the most prominent Black officials in the federal government, his was a welcome lone voice of conscience.

Perhaps the most zealous in trying to deny mistreatment in the name of unity was (also Black) Washington, D.C., mayor Anthony Williams:

> It would be another victory for the terrorists if in one aftermath of all this that you've got one group of public servants—postal employees, who are doing their job—pointing fingers at another group of public servants—the people at the Centers for Disease Control, who are just humbly trying

to do their job. The last thing I think that they would want to do is try to discriminate between groups providing treatment.[56]

Although Williams is correct that notions of a racist conspiracy among CDC employees would be unfounded, conscious malevolence is not really what critics were alleging. On the contrary, the routine and thoughtless nature of the disparities makes them more appalling, not less. Trying to brush deadly inequality under the rug of American worker unity leads to my final concern, what Amy Alexander has termed the "whitewashing of terror." Again from Mayor Williams:

> These attacks in our country are indiscriminate. They really know no income lines, they know no class lines, they know no racial lines, they know no denomination lines. Whoever these people are, are attacking people irrespective of where they're from or what they believe.[57]

On a certain level, Mayor Williams's protestations are completely true. The various terrorists involved in both the September 11 attacks and the anthrax crisis certainly did not have a particular desire to kill African Americans, working class or otherwise. (In all likelihood, the anthrax terrorist didn't want to kill anyone—hence the clear warnings accompanying the anthrax of what it was and how to medicate those exposed.) On the contrary, well-heeled white men were apparently the main targets of both rounds of terrorism and the suffering of others a secondary effect. But Williams is sidestepping the legitimate concerns of D.C.'s Black postal workers, which have less to do with conspiracies by terrorists or by governments than with the way in which a supposedly united America continues both to render African Americans' suffering invisible and to protect African Americans less.

Amy Alexander, who wrote "Bleaching the Disaster" a week before these postal workers became ill, coined the phrase "whitewashing of terror" to describe what she noticed in the dediversification of images of terror victims and heroes.[58] She argues that in the immediate coverage of September 11, television and print images were being put out so fast that they looked just as New York does—profoundly multicultural. But as time went on and editing increased, the picture of New York started to look more and more like what Erna Smith has called "Woody Allen's New York": all white. (The notable exception was the *New York Times,* which published *all* the victims' pictures and biographical sketches.)

Although the television images could not help but reveal the postal workers' race, the newspapers need not do so. Typically, they did not.[59] The newspaper references that came up on LexisNexis for "black AND postal worker" were from Canada and Britain. Those newspapers had quotes from postal workers that were completely unlike what the American press had reported, for example, from the London *Daily Telegraph*:

> "I think it's racial," said Gail Saxton, 48, who sorted post in the express mail room alongside Leroy Richmond, one of the two victims recovering in hospital. "I hate to say it, but it's a fact. We lost two members of the postal family and that wasn't necessary." Last week, she said, she had been forced to buy her own gloves and face mask because her managers refused to supply them. "They did us a raw deal. They closed Capitol Hill down completely. But all they were telling us was 'You gotta get out the mail.' There was no concern for people like us. It's terrible, but it's been going on for years. It's nothing new. Yeah, I'm an American. I feel glad to be one. But we know that as African-Americans we are treated as second-class citizens."[60]

This worker's words contrast starkly with the many postal workers' quotes included in the U.S. press and with the editorials written, which talked about "the little people" getting mistreated without identifying them as nonwhite.[61] It is possible that the more far-flung newspaper editorialists did not even know that "the little people" in question were Black, since none of the dominant print news sources—the *New York Times,* the *Washington Post,* and the wire services—had identified them as such. If they did know, the columnists could have been appropriating the suffering of these men as their own (as fellow Americans and fellow little people), or they could have been doing just what the national news sources were: making conscious decisions not to emphasize race despite how the event was being experienced on the ground.

Being local to the disaster, the *Washington Post* could not avoid at least mentioning concerns about racism in its conciliatory summing up of the events: "complaints were rising that officials had acted less swiftly to defend the blue-collar, often minority workers of the Postal Service than they had the white-collar, mainly white world of Capitol Hill. A close examination of the events of that week suggests that Brentwood workers were not victims of such a double standard."[62] The *Post* does not mention the race of those minority workers, nor that of the victims. The phrase "often minority" serves as a gross understatement. No pictures accompany the article.

In contrast with the mainstream press, the Black press in D.C. and elsewhere (while woefully short on giving voice to the postal workers) was very clear in its implication of race in the disparity:

> The double standards of life in America are hard to overlook, especially when one group historically becomes the victims. Television exposed the reality that the Senate Office Buildings, where most of the employees are white, received a quick response to the potentially deadly anthrax threat. On the other hand, employees who initially handled the mail sent to Sen. Daschle's office, from a location often referred to as "the Plantation" and who are predominantly black, were overlooked, an oversight that may have contributed to the death of two postal employees and the infection of several others.[63]

Amy Alexander, who had raised concerns about the whitewashing of terror, also wrote about the refusal to see these victims as Black. She takes issue with Postmaster General John E. "Jack" Potter's statement that "this is not a situation where Americans should be pointing fingers at anyone else other than the terrorists":

> His comments were a clear effort to diffuse black postal workers' complaints that they had been shafted. But for me they simply raise new fears that all the psychic energy we are now expending on the war effort, and all the material sacrifices we are being called on to make, will be particularly burdensome for people who have for centuries given their all with little help or return from our government.[64]

Alexander is also concerned that one result of the lack of adequate treatment for postal workers will be that it "will feed into longstanding fears held by many blacks that the government's health services systems might abuse (through neglect or action) African Americans." For my part, I believe that those fears are grounded and necessary. Increased skepticism would not be a negative outcome if it could allow more people to get care like that Leroy Richmond received.

The *Journal of the American Medical Association,* which often does mention the race of patients, did not in these cases: they are described as "a 47-year-old male postal worker who worked in the mail sorting area of the Brentwood facility" and "a 55-year-old male postal worker who worked as a distribution clerk in the mail sorting area of the Brentwood facility and who had hypertension, diabetes mellitus, and remote history of sarcoidosis."[65] We might simply attribute the absence of race here by noting that race is not relevant to the diagnosis—but it is not clear how gender or exact age is, either. It would be perfectly routine to include "black" between the age and the gender. Although not much can be said definitively about the absence of a descriptor, it might well have something to do with the history of medical interest in comparative racial pathology, which has sought answers that are based in biology rather than in politics.[66] The routine inclusion of race in medical histories neither historically nor today generally seeks what progressives might want it to, which is to indict inadequate care.[67]

The resistance in the media to recognizing the differential impact of anthrax on a Black population comes in part, I think, from an allegiance to the particular narrative developed by President George W. Bush and others that pronounced the events of September 11 as an attack on civilization or on the values of freedom itself. Recognizing our own civilization as imperfect at such a moment led to being criticized for undermining that thing for which we were fighting.

Anthropologist Veena Das provides valuable insights into the aspects of America that must be obscured to maintain unquestioned faith in an uncomplicatedly just and democratic America. "What these statements conjure is the idea of the United States . . . as embodying these values—not contingently, not as a horizon in relation to struggles within its borders against, say, slavery, racism, or the destruction of native American populations, but as if a teleology has particularly privileged it to embody these values."[68] To maintain this fiction of a unified America "as the privileged site of universal values," Das points out that along the way, "representations of the American nation manage to obscure from view the experiences of those within its body politics who were never safe even before September 11."[69]

> OPERATOR: If there's anything, if your condition starts to worsen, have your wife give us a call back, OK?
> MORRIS: All right.
> OPERATOR: All right then.
> MORRIS: Thank you.

Wishful thinking about government and medical response to terror is dangerous. Trust was fatal for Morris and Curseen, and skepticism saved Richmond. As Jill Nelson writes:

> we want to believe that as American citizens, we are all in this together, as equals. We want to believe that the government knows what it is doing. We do not want to believe the worst, even though we have experienced it before: That race and class, fame and fortune would inform the response to this crisis. . . . But it's way past time we as Americans realized that wishing doesn't make it so.[70]

Indeed, Black men, including these postal workers, have never been safe in the United States. Underscoring the ways in which the medical and political systems fail them may disrupt the fantasy of a perfect America, but that disruption is necessary if the protection that purports to be provided is to be truly extended to all.

2

Un/natural Disaster

CHRONIC DISEASE AFTER HURRICANE KATRINA

Hurricane Katrina hit southeast Louisiana in late August 2005.[1] The storm made its first landfall in Florida on Thursday, August 25, and weakened briefly as it passed overland before it reached the Gulf of Mexico on Friday, August 26, where it quickly strengthened over the warm water. The storm's second landfall came early in the morning on Monday, August 29, near the Louisiana–Mississippi border. That day and the next, the levees that protected New Orleans failed, and 80 percent of the city was flooded—mostly residential areas. The mortality count is still contested, but more than seventeen hundred people were killed, and hundreds of thousands were displaced.[2]

The fact that a hurricane is a natural disaster might create an intuitive sense that its harms might be random, but that is far from the case. Hurricane Katrina's impacts were unnaturally distributed, exacerbating preexisting inequalities.[3] In 2005, New Orleans was a socially and culturally vibrant but profoundly unequal city, in which the legacies of centuries of slavery and legally enforced segregation were palpable. The impacts of the storm were most heavily borne by New Orleans residents who were Black and poor.

In the initial days after the storm, as mass media was captivated by wildly overblown and unfounded notions that survivors faced extreme danger of violence from other survivors, there was a great deal of worry among public health experts about the spread of infectious disease. For public health authorities, the concerns were about wound infections and waterborne gastrointestinal diseases such as cholera as sanitation infrastructures were flooded, as well as mosquito-borne diseases.[4] For lay publics, the presence of dead bodies in the water seemed manifestly dangerous to survivors' health.[5] The squalid conditions in the temporary shelters of the Superdome and the Convention Center, which quickly lost plumbing and air conditioning and so were rife with putrefying human waste, seemed like obvious circumstances for an infectious disease outbreak. And yet it became clear even during the initial emergency, and certainly within weeks of the storm, that for those who survived the flooding itself, it was *chronic disease*—especially cardiovascular disease—that emerged as a far greater contributor to excess morbidity and mortality.[6] This health impact is far less obvious: how can a flood cause chronic disease?

A crisis on the scale of Hurricane Katrina might contribute to chronic disease in many ways, including through stress.[7] Especially in the days and weeks after the storm's landfall, psychosocial stress was a key contributor to a spike in cardiovascular events and cardiovascular disease hospitalizations—a phenomenon that was particularly pronounced among African Americans, as long-standing cardiovascular disease disparities were exacerbated.[8] In the first six months after the storm, the significant increase in the mortality rate has been attributed to the compromised public health infrastructure that was not able to identify and address the population's health problems.[9] Yet the increase in the incidence of such health problems as acute myocardial infarction (heart attack) continued for at least ten years after the storm and has many causes.[10]

In this chapter, I attend to ways in which the unnatural disaster of this storm played a role in increased chronic disease. I focus especially on how the multifaceted structural exclusion of Katrina victims from full membership in the U.S. body politic intersected with one particular, tangible element of lack of access to health care: pharmaceuticals. Focusing on pharmaceuticals is analytically helpful because, as anthropologists of pharmaceuticals have pointed out, drugs help to make dis-ease concrete.[11] That is, pharmaceuticals can help to make tangible the distress in the body and in the society that might otherwise be hard to pin down.

I track the travels of pharmaceuticals in the aftermath of Hurricane Katrina to explore three key ways in which the response to the emergency exacerbated the preexisting vulnerability of the population, especially with regard to health: at emergency shelters, in drug donation programs, and in ongoing care. Each of these disrupted pharmaceutical flows provides an opportunity to see ways that those most acutely impacted by Hurricane Katrina were framed as outside of the "mainstream American public," in intertwining ways: as criminals, as refugees, and as marginalized. Disrupted pharmaceutical flows at emergency shelters exemplify ways in which Katrina victims were impacted by discourses and practices associated with criminality; disrupted pharmaceutical flows in drug donation programs do the same with regard to global health complexes; and disrupted pharmaceutical flows in ongoing care illuminate their marginalization. Being outside ordinary pharmaceutical flows and being outside the "American public" occur through mutually reinforcing processes. These processes illustrate pathways by which racial inequality becomes materially embodied.

I conclude with discussion of how this case illustrates racialized biopolitics, with reference to philosopher Michel Foucault's influential introduction of the idea of biopolitics in his "Society Must Be Defended."[12] In a Foucauldian biopolitics in which power fosters (some) life and lets (other) life die, being ideologically defined as outside of society is intertwined with being materially left for dead.

ACUTE DISRUPTION OF FLOWS: CRIMINALIZATION AT THE SUPERDOME AND ACROSS THE CITY

The most acute disruption of the flow of pharmaceuticals happened in the immediate aftermath of the storm, when the city was still largely underwater. One poignant story that I heard about events at the Superdome, where twenty thousand or more people who were trapped in New Orleans found squalid shelter from the flood,[13] provides an analytical entry point. There were and are many rumors and conflicting accounts about what happened at the Superdome, and it is difficult to be definitive, and yet one physician's account that I heard at a conference provides an evocative frame.

The context was the American College of Cardiology (ACC) meeting in New Orleans in 2007, which drew thousands of cardiologists and other health care providers to the city. The meeting had been scheduled long before Katrina and would be the first large conference held in New Orleans after the storm.[14] These kinds of meetings usually feel rather placeless, a series of science-driven panels in interchangeable conference rooms with perhaps one or two panels of "local relevance." But that entire ACC meeting felt inescapably aware of the deeply damaged city outside. The Association of Black Cardiologists sponsored a panel about Hurricane Katrina within the larger conference, and the experience of attending this "local relevance" panel has stayed with me.

At the panel, one of the local doctors who had gone to the Superdome to help serve his displaced patients gave a harrowing account. He said that the National Guard troops stationed at the Superdome had been instructed not to allow people seeking shelter there to bring in drugs—including pharmaceuticals outside of their original packaging. Some unknown amount of prescription drugs was confiscated and discarded. By the time the physician arrived on the scene, he had to try to reconstruct complex prescription regimens of elderly, distressed patients, from their memories.

I have not been able to track down much documentation for this story, and I do not know how widely followed this National Guard practice was. That said, it is a scandal at whatever scope. The National Guard practice that this physician described was clearly a policy informed by the War on Drugs, and it prioritized restricting access to illicit drugs at the expense of access to licit ones. In this practice at the Superdome, enforcing drug policies framed the racialized population of Katrina's survivors not as members of the community in need of care but as potential criminals in need of control.[15]

Selective control of drugs and social control of Black people have long had intertwined histories in the United States.[16] The War on Drugs is itself a central mechanism of ongoing racial inequality. As legal scholar Michelle Alexander has influentially argued, the War on Drugs is central to a contemporary system of racial control, even as it formally adheres to "color-blindness."[17] Since those with criminal convictions can be treated as less than full citizens, and since such convictions track not illicit drug use (which occurs at similar rates in all racial groups) but rather exposure to the criminal justice system, drug laws can become a way of disenfranchising whole communities—especially those that are predominantly Black and poor. In this physician's account of what happened at the Superdome, those seeking refuge were treated as presumptive enemies in the drug war.

This particular element of the disruption of pharmaceutical flows at the Superdome was consistent with the broader ways in which *criminal* tropes were invoked to describe Katrina's displaced people in the immediate aftermath of the storm.[18] Within two days of the storm, when many people were still awaiting rescue, the multiple levels of government (city, state, federal) were already explicitly shifting priorities from saving lives to imposing order. As political scientist Melissa Harris-Perry has argued, "for black Americans the disastrous consequences of wind and water were deepened by the initially slow and then surprisingly militaristic response to black suffering."[19] In the progressive magazine the *Nation,* journalist Rebecca Solnit quoted a news report from the Associated Press on September 1, in which the mayor ordered fifteen hundred police officers "to leave their search-and-rescue mission Wednesday night and return to the streets of the beleaguered city to stop looting that has turned increasingly hostile."[20] She elaborated, "Only two days after the catastrophe struck, while thousands were still stuck on roofs, in attics, on overpasses, on second and third stories and in isolated buildings on high ground in flooded neighborhoods, the mayor chose protecting property over human life."[21]

The restoration of social order was explicitly not defined as restoration of services and infrastructure but as the restoration of punishment for property crime.[22] There were explicit articulations from authorities that "law and order" would have to be established *before* relief agencies such as the Red Cross could do their work. This resonates with the account of the actions of the National Guard at the Superdome, putting drug control ahead of public health.

The mass media intensified the articulation of those impacted by the hurricane as criminals. From the start, survivors were described as "marauding" and, most widely, "looting." Whereas searching for food amid the debris of abandoned supermarkets might be understood to be a perfectly logical thing for a storm victim to do, the poor and Black people left behind in New Orleans were routinely described as "looting." As

Kathleen Tierney and colleagues observe in their analysis of media coverage of disasters, "in Katrina's aftermath, among the most widely circulated media images was a set of photographs in which African Americans were consistently described as 'looting' goods, while whites engaging in exactly the same behaviors were labeled as 'finding' supplies."[23] This is of a piece with the broader and profoundly racialized characterization of Katrina victims as engaging in behavior typical of riots, rather than natural disasters.[24] In riots, looting is indeed common and complexly socially condoned, though we should also question the media obsession with looting during rebellions against racial injustice.[25] But the assumption that this particular community could only be antisocial in the context of crisis rendered invisible the broadly prosocial behavior that people displaced by the storm undertook—helping each other.[26] The dominant framing of Katrina victims was as subhuman, lacking basic human decency, rather than as community members, much less citizens.

In response to the threat of property crimes, Louisiana governor Kathleen Blanco gave chilling shoot-to-kill orders, which were widely reported: "These troops are fresh back from Iraq, well trained, experienced, battle tested and under my orders to restore order in the streets. They have M-16s and they are locked and loaded. These troops know how to shoot and kill and they are more than willing to do so if necessary and I expect they will."[27] Even within the military response, there was dissent to this approach, as Lieutenant General Russel Honoré, Joint Task Force commander who was also a Louisiana native, attempted to set a different tone, pleading with troops: "Imagine being rescued and having a fellow American point a gun at you. These are Americans. This is not Iraq."[28] Yet even this protestation reinforces the sense that this space was understood within the frame of a war zone, not the United States.

Conventionally, there is a jurisdictional gap in domain between police forces, who are meant to protect citizens, and military forces, who are meant to enforce sovereign territorial power, but this contrast doesn't fully hold. And during Katrina, we see the involvement of military enforcement side by side with police enforcement to protect property rather than people. This is a theme that will be relevant in later chapters as well, especially on the Flint water crisis: when it comes to people whose claim to citizenship is tenuous, property can easily outrank them in the priorities of the state.

At emergency shelters like the Superdome, as throughout the city, the survivors left behind were not afforded a presumption of innocence, as citizens to protect rather than criminals to control. The ideological criminalization—the criminal-infested city prone to urban riot—framed those affected by the storm as "un-American." The enrollment of military personnel pointed toward an additional frame, which was the "war zone." This, in turn, connects both to the profound othering of the victims that the criminalization rhetorics provided and to the chapter's next theme: "refugees."

INAPPROPRIATE FLOWS: INADEQUATE STOCKPILES
AND DONATIONS FOR "REFUGEES"

The flows of pharmaceuticals in the subsequent days and weeks were also revealing. The governmental emergency stockpiles of pharmaceuticals did not match Katrina victims' needs, and programs put in place to donate drugs didn't either. Whether the overwhelmingly Black and poor communities impacted were truly part of the American public was again at stake. Whereas those seeking provisions in the flooded city and shelter at the Superdome were framed as outside the mainstream American public through rhetorics of criminalization, those in need of care in the days and weeks that followed were framed as outside of the mainstream public through rhetorics of "refugees."

As with the othering language of "looters," the othering language of "refugees" is also worth paying attention to. The term *refugee* was widely used during the peak of the crisis, even as it was pointedly contested by survivors who objected that they were not refugees but "American citizens with rights."[29] We might problematize the stigmatization of refugees on which this demand to be excepted from the category implies, but it does important work. As Tulane University anthropologist Adeline Masquelier observes, reflecting on her own journey as well as those of her fellow New Orleans residents, "the word 'refugee,' as this war on words suggests, carries a heavy semantic load."[30]

The refugee is a more sympathetic figure than the criminal—and the figuration of refugees as sympathetic was far stronger in 2005 than it would become later in the fifteen years between Hurricane Katrina and this writing—but the refugee is still not part of the public.[31] Help for the refugee is at the whim of the secure occupant. The ways that pharmaceuticals flowed show that Katrina refugees were positioned in ways analogous to the Global South citizens who are the targets of the Global Health Complex—a philanthropically driven system in which efforts to address the needs of the world's poor operate in the service of heterogeneous private interests.[32] Indeed, international nongovernmental organizations that typically provide services in the Global South became part of the chaotic network of those involved in Katrina relief. For example, the international humanitarian organization Oxfam, which focuses on alleviating poverty—its name derives from the Oxford Committee for Famine Relief, though its scope is now more broad—rarely addresses humanitarian crises on U.S. soil but made an exception for Hurricane Katrina.[33]

Medicines for chronic disease are not typically thought of as part of emergency provisions, at the household level or the system level. At hospitals and clinics serving Katrina evacuees, these drugs were not to hand. Fred Cerise, secretary of the Louisiana Department of Health and Hospitals, would testify in federal Senate hearings about the impact of Katrina:

> Another area that we were challenged in, again having to do with people with chronic disease, was access to pharmaceuticals. Again, traditionally in public health disasters we think about things like having access to biologicals and things, antidotes for biological weapons, and that sort of medicine stockpile that is available. The stockpile we needed was the stockpile of medicines for blood pressure and diabetes and heart disease and things like that.[34]

Treatment for chronic conditions was a major driver of those seeking care from emergency medical treatment sites in the weeks after the storm.[35] Yet these gaps in the institutional stockpiles meant that even those storm survivors who managed to carry individual backup supplies quickly ran out, and this had a serious impact on those fleeing Hurricane Katrina, especially those who were old and frail.[36]

Donations were coming into shelters and community health centers from heterogeneous sources and were chaotically uncoordinated. A physician reporting about preparations at the Superdome in the lead-up to the storm wrote:

> At that time, the [National] Guard had trucks moving supplies of weapons (for security), bottled water and MREs (meals ready to eat) into the same loading dock, which we had full of patients. Supplies came in by the thousands—four 18-wheel truckloads of bottled water and two loads of MREs. But no one brought in standard medical supplies, such as medications for hypertension, diabetes, asthma or other chronic diseases.[37]

One ad hoc pharmacy opened by Public Health Service staff in a federal medical station received a limited number of drugs from the Strategic National Stockpile, but that supply was determined by particular expectations of disaster and included, for example, little insulin and no tetanus vaccines.[38] This pharmaceutical portfolio problem has been recognized in global health research as well, as researchers have advocated inclusion of pharmaceuticals for noncommunicable diseases in the standard emergency health kit.[39] And yet the global health paradigm's focus on infectious disease is pervasive, and this mind-set combined with resource constraints means that it is hard to effect change.

Donation programs are a common way of dealing with crises and are inadequate. Like similar programs in the realm of global health, drug donation programs provided some essential relief during Katrina, but they were inefficient, and their provisions were often inappropriate. There was a mismatch between the medication provisions that the disaster medical teams stocked for treatment of the storm's victims and their medication needs, such that many evacuees had to rely on retail pharmacies for their chronic disease treatments.[40] The mismatch is a way in which the experience of Katrina mirrors problems in global health: pharmaceutical companies love to tout their generosity in their public relations campaigns, but drug donation programs do not necessarily serve the needs of patients.[41]

Community health providers serving Katrina survivors observed:

> Although providers received helpful donations of medications, many—
> often cut off from communication channels—reported receiving large
> quantities of unrequested, inappropriate, and expired medications from
> unidentified sources. Classifying medications and disposing of unusable
> items was a burden on providers already struggling to dispose of disaster-
> related debris. In some instances, providers were forced to let surpluses
> become ruined in inclement weather due to lack of storage space.[42]

In their reliance on inadequate pharmaceutical donation programs, we can
see that Katrina's survivors were situated more similarly to those in poor
countries than those in the United States. In the social science literature
critical of "pharmaceuticalization," there has been a widespread bifurcation
between analysts of the Global North, who focus on "disease mongering"
and overprescribing, and analysts of the Global South, who focus on access programs and the inadequacy of framing access to pharmaceuticals
(iconically antiretrovirals) as access to health.[43]

Yet with regard to coronary artery disease therapeutics in the United
States, analytical focus on excessive treatment driven by pharmaceutical industry interests has obscured attention to deep stratification:
overtreatment in some populations and undertreatment in others, along
economic and racialized lines.[44] This extends beyond prescription rates to
the physical possession of pharmaceuticals—with Black people less likely
than white people to live in a household in which all members requiring
medication have a three-day supply to hand in case of an emergency.[45]
Pharmaceuticals to avert the risk of cardiovascular disease are famously
pervasive in the United States[46]—and yet the citizens most impacted by
Katrina were left out.

Writing several months after Katrina, a group of authors from the
Centers for Disease Control and Prevention urged collection of baseline
chronic disease data in populations to help disaster preparedness, and
yet observed:

> Little has been published about treating chronically ill people during
> disasters. Perhaps this is because many of the disasters have occurred in

poor countries where chronic disease has been historically less of a health priority. Or perhaps in wealthier countries, catastrophic damage to the medical infrastructure is uncommon, so patients with chronic diseases continue to receive care.[47]

In this sense, there is a profound connection between un-American-ness and being figured as a recipient of classic emergency response, and Katrina victims found themselves on the wrong side of that insider–outsider divide.

Anxieties about infectious disease might be fundamental enough to emergency management that we might not see that focus as racialized. However, the association between Blackness and those most vulnerable to emergency is also meaningful. Blackness itself has long been associated with infectious disease rather than chronic disease, and that association has a very long history in the United States. Chronic diseases—especially cancer and heart disease—are seen as "diseases of modernity," and states of emergency and Blackness both put modernity into question.[48] There has long been a tension between the idea that "germs know no color line" and the idea that there is an association between Blackness and infectiousness.[49] The "imagined communities" of belonging carry with them "imagined immunities," such that only those outside "normal conditions" of "the mainstream public" are figured as vulnerable to premodern infectious diseases.[50]

There are international laws regarding the treatment and rights of refugees, but these are widely violated. Refugees have more modest entitlements than full citizens, and being subject to the whims of those who tolerate them, and what they are willing to provide to them, is part of the constitution of their vulnerability. Even though it is the case that access to needed pharmaceuticals would not by itself resolve the marginalization of those impacted by Katrina,[51] their exclusion from access still flags exclusion from the body politic. That Katrina victims found themselves in this structural and semantic position outside the "American public" exemplifies their unjustly incomplete citizenship.

PRECARIOUS FLOWS: A FRAGILE SAFETY NET TORN

There is a third set of disruptions of pharmaceutical flows to attend to: the disruption of already tenuous continuity of care left many patients without knowledge of, much less access to, their prior pharmaceutical treatment regimens. It is very easy for barely managed diabetes to become unmanaged diabetes, for barely managed heart failure to become unmanaged heart failure. In chronic disease, as in life more generally, those who are close to the edge are made still more vulnerable in a crisis.

Six months after the storm, the medical providers working in the diminished number of hospitals still operational in New Orleans were confronted with serious complications of unmet chronic health care needs. The chief medical officer of West Jefferson Medical Center noted, "These people come in with extremely severe problems. Diabetics have been off their insulin for six months. They come to us in diabetic ketoacidosis."[52] Since Hurricane Katrina, there has been increasing recognition of the role of chronic disease in disaster's impacts. However, this too often leads to individual-level recommendations—for example, "a focus on personal preparedness for people with NCDs [noncommunicable diseases]."[53] That is, the responsibility falls on the chronically ill individual to prepare, rather than on the state to construct resilient systems.

Before the storm, the vulnerable populations of New Orleans had largely relied on the city's public hospital system, rather than on personal physicians. A bit of context can help to understand how this matters. In the United States, the public hospital system has never been "public" in the same sense as, for example, the National Health Service in the United Kingdom, which serves everyone. Instead, it was set up specifically for the indigent. New Orleans's Charity Hospital was founded in the eighteenth century primarily to serve white immigrants and would later serve all New Orleanians on a segregated basis in the era of Jim Crow.[54] Although the civil rights movement would end official de jure segregation at the hospital, like many such integrated institutions, it became de facto segregated as it was largely abandoned by white patients. The hospital struggled to meet its mission of serving all those in need of care, which includes those without health insurance.

Charity Hospital was the central node of the safety network on which New Orleans residents relied, and it weathered the storm poorly. It was permanently closed a month after the storm, to the alarm of human rights advocates concerned that those who had relied on it had nowhere else to turn in the private and piecemeal terrain of care that replaced the landmark hospital.[55] As analysts who interviewed Katrina survivors who had relocated to Houston observed, "with Charity hospital destroyed, so were the medical records and any hope of continuity of health care for these individuals. In contrast, individuals who have health insurance coverage at the time of a crisis can access care more easily in another setting or location."[56] When the hospital system was decimated, so was these Katrina survivors' access to care.

Because the care provided by underfunded hospitals like Charity was not necessarily up to par with care elsewhere, some might imagine that the private system that has replaced it would be less racist and provide higher-quality outcomes—but the abandonment of marginalized communities has only intensified in the new system.[57] Those who have public health insurance can in principle use those resources to access the private system. That includes the state-based system of Medicaid, for the poor and disabled, and the national system of Medicare, for those age sixty-five and older. But like the New Orleans public school system that has been replaced with a publicly funded private charter system, the liberal model of education and health care for all that had been falling short for many was replaced with an education and health care system reconstructed along neoliberal models that intensified exclusions.[58] Whereas the public institutions of liberal democracy have long failed to fully serve citizens who are Black and poor, market-driven neoliberal replacements for state services are not the escape that they pretend to be.

For people living in precarity, long-term risk-reducing drugs might be less pressing than other concerns, and this is even more true in the context of emergency and major life disruption. Even when patients had prescriptions, they didn't necessarily have the means to fill them in the places in which they found refuge. And whether they remained in New Orleans or joined the far-flung diaspora, many had no clear place to turn for help. In one telephone survey of a geographically representative sample of Katrina survivors, investigators found that 73.9 percent of respondents reported having one or more chronic conditions in the year before the hurricane and that one-fifth (20.6 percent) had had their treatment disrupted.[59] Of course, as the authors acknowledge, phone surveys likely undercount the sickest and most unstable of the total target population, and yet the results are still informative. Common reasons for disruption included lack of health insurance and residential instability. Those too young to qualify for Medicare, which as a national program is portable across the United States, were more likely to stop treatment.[60] This disruption to the care of the relatively young points to the potential for very long-standing impacts of the disruptions of the storm, as those who forgo risk-reducing pharmaceuticals at that age come to experience increased morbidity and mortality impacts later on.

It is difficult to make comprehensive claims about the precise statistics of long-term cardiovascular and other chronic disease impacts on Katrina victims because of the dispersion of that population. But studies at particular sites are stark. For example, at Tulane University Health Sciences Center in downtown New Orleans, there was a threefold increase in admissions for acute myocardial infarction (heart attack) documented two years poststorm[61] and again six years after the storm.[62] Even ten years after the storm, there were no signs of heart attack rates returning to prestorm levels.[63]

The more chronic elements of this lack of treatment for chronic disease illustrate something fundamental about the ways that emergencies exacerbate existing inequalities. There is a resonance here with rhetorics of terrorism after September 11 discussed in the previous chapter, which misleadingly framed Americans as newly vulnerable. As geographer Susan Cutter observes, "the revelations of inadequate response to the hurricane's aftermath are not just about failures in emergency response at the local, state, and federal levels or failures in the overall emergency management system. They are also about failures of the social support systems for America's impoverished—the largely invisible inner city poor."[64]

CONCLUSION: IF SOCIETY MUST BE DEFENDED, RACIALIZED POPULATIONS ARE OFTEN LEFT OUT

If many Americans could treat the devastation in New Orleans as intruding on nostalgia for a beautiful historical city and raucous "party town," for the disproportionately Black and poor communities who had lived there, Hurricane Katrina marked an intensification of already existing exclusions and vulnerability.[65] The impact of this marginalization has been borne in their hearts, not just in a metaphorical sense, but literally, as even more than a decade later, they continue to suffer greater burdens of heart disease. The etiology of this heart disease, as of chronic disease more broadly, importantly includes, even as it exceeds, the impact of insufficient access to pharmaceuticals.

An editorial published a month after the storm in the *British Medical Journal* by authors from a U.S. governmental research center on health disparities describes the shock of media images of Hurricane Katrina's immediate aftermath: "Live images of uncollected corpses and families clinging to rooftops made vivid what decades of statistics could not: that being poor in America, and especially being poor and black in a poor southern state, is still hazardous to your health."[66] Yet they overstate the contrast between this event and the routine when they write:

> This may truly be a "teachable moment" about the impact of poverty and race on health. The gap in health between white and black Americans has been estimated to cause 84,000 excess deaths a year in the United States, a virtual Katrina every week. Because the victims gradually succumb to various diseases such as diabetes, cardiovascular disease, alcohol and drug abuse, cancer, and HIV infection, they rarely capture the public's attention in the way the victims of Katrina have. As a result, health inequality has persisted despite decades of important health gains, economic growth, and progress on racial issues in the United States.[67]

But as we have seen in this chapter, the impact of Katrina extends beyond the acute moments of being stranded on rooftops. The storm's aftermath includes and intensifies all of these mechanisms of ordinary health disparities.

In the wake of Katrina, we see a stark instantiation of biopolitics in Michel Foucault's sense. The name given to the set of lectures in which he introduced the concept is itself evocative: "Society Must Be Defended."[68] If society must be defended, who is in, and who is out?

The building and maintenance of the infrastructure of cities is a fundamental aspect of biopolitics, and the failure of infrastructure after Katrina illuminates its operation. Consider the meaning of biopower: Foucault argues that if, in premodern times, sovereignty was exercised by taking people's lives or letting them live, modern power would now also operate by making people live and letting them die.[69] This happens not just at the level of individuals but also in aggregates, including with regard to the engineering of environments. Foucault notes that "this includes the direct effects of the geographical, climatic, or hydrographic environment: the problem, for instance, of swamps"[70]—so important in shaping New Orleans. "And also the problem of the environment to the extent that it is not a natural environment, that it has been created by the population and therefore has effects on that population. This is, essentially, the urban problem."[71] The infrastructure of New Orleans was meant to foster life in the city—but for some more than others.

If the infrastructure was built to differentially foster life, in the aftermath of its failure, the inaction in the face of need intensified inequities in ways that are also revealing. The operation of racism is at stake. In his lecture, Foucault is interested in the connection between biopolitics and racism in a different sense, of eugenics, of "purifying the race"—as exemplified most starkly in Nazi Germany's extermination of those groups of people who were considered to be biologically inferior.[72] Foucault points out that the biopolitics of fostering the life of those who are legitimately part of the society can be a justification for killing those who are not. But even when racism is warlike, as when enforced by the National Guard, it is not necessarily eugenic. A racist biopolitics need not be eugenic to have racially disparate deadly impacts. Hurricane Katrina and its aftermath are emblematic of a biopolitics of racism that operates by defining who is and is not part of the society that must be defended. The most pervasive element of the racialized control of life and death is enacted, not by killing those considered to be outside of and a threat to society, but by neglecting to foster the lives of those considered to be less than full members of society.[73]

This chapter builds on the previous one not just chronologically but analytically as well. Some analysts have put the suffering of Katrina explicitly into the context of post-9/11 America, in which political goals took precedence over authentic disaster preparedness.[74] In neither case did crisis spur investment in or engagement with addressing chronic health inequalities. As political scientist Melissa Harris-Perry has argued, "the entire nation grieved over the losses in New Orleans, but for black America, the aftermath of Hurricane Katrina forced the question of whether black people were truly American citizens worthy of fair treatment, swift response, and unchallenged rescue."[75]

In the days, weeks, and years that have followed, tracking pharmaceutical travels reveals how (lack of) access to medicines reflected (lack of) access to citizenship and health for the racialized population impacted by Hurricane Katrina and its aftermath. As the next chapter turns to more explicitly biopolitical questions of "biological citizenship" that come to the fore in the structure of mass incarceration, this fundamental question of the racialization of American citizenship in its broadest senses remains inescapable.

3

Mass Incarceration

ON THE SUSPENDED SENTENCES
OF THE SCOTT SISTERS

On December 29, 2010, Mississippi governor Haley Barbour suspended the dual life sentences of two African American sisters who had spent sixteen years in prison, imposing an extraordinary condition: that Gladys Scott donate a kidney to her ailing sister, Jamie Scott. Close attention to the event and the context of Governor Barbour's decision to make prison release contingent upon organ donation helps to situate mass incarceration as a key site of the contemporary biopolitics of racism.

Though not as high profile as many of the other cases discussed in this book, the plight of the Scott sisters had been a rallying point for both mainstream and radical civil rights advocates, and the Scott sisters' conditional release garnered commentary both from civil rights advocates who had long sought the sisters' release[1] and from bioethicists and critical legal scholars.[2] This chapter attends to the Scott sisters case in light of the broader critique of mass incarceration as a structurally racist institution and in light of how prison imposes biological control on prisoners—both in ordinary circumstances, by structuring access to health care, and in extraordinary circumstances, such as organ donation schemes. The biomedical process of organ donation renders particular relations visible, and my analysis puts different models of biological citizenship and therapeutic citizenship into relief to highlight the specificity of the U.S. context of famously high-tech medicine and infamously unequal access to care.

SISTERS UNJUSTLY INCARCERATED, INSPIRING
A CAMPAIGN FOR RELEASE

Jamie and Gladys Scott were young mothers aged nineteen and twenty-one without previous criminal records when they were charged with a role in a December 1993 robbery in Forest, Mississippi. The sisters do not speak about the case, but according to the transcript of the criminal trial, they allegedly lured two male acquaintances into a secluded area, where three other men, who were armed, struck them with a gun and robbed them of their wallets.³ No one was hurt, and the robbery has been widely reported to have netted only eleven dollars.⁴ Two of the three young men who were convicted of actually doing the armed robbery testified against the sisters as part of plea bargains in exchange for reduced sentences, and all three of the men served fewer than three years.⁵ Although even the prosecutor in the case has described it as "not a particularly egregious case," the sisters were convicted in October 1994 and given extraordinary sentences: double life.⁶

Jamie Scott wrote a pamphlet from prison about their case in 2003, in what would mark the beginning of a long campaign. She credited "the voice of God" as inspiration and described praying while she typed.⁷ Their mother, Evelyn Rasco, started a blog to publicize the pamphlet and, later, to coordinate protests.⁸ As in a great deal of prison organizing, faith and family intertwined: according to a reporter for Jackson's African American newspaper the *Jackson Advocate,* the Scott family showed "the power of a God-fearing family."⁹ Mainstream and radical civil rights organizations campaigned for the sisters as well, including the NAACP and the Malcolm X Grassroots Movement.¹⁰ The inspiring Black nationalist lawyer and city council member who would later become the mayor of Jackson, Chokwe Lumumba, played an important role.¹¹

Fifteen years into their imprisonment, organizing around the sisters' case was gaining strength, but their bodies were very weakened: demands for their release became particularly urgent in January 2010, when Jamie went into end-stage kidney failure. According to a flyer for a fundraiser for the sisters, medical maltreatment in prison had caused the health crisis and, in the absence of adequate care, "Jamie Scott has now effectively been sentenced to death."[12] Gladys volunteered to donate a kidney to her sister and stipulated as much in a petition for pardon submitted on the sisters' behalf by Chokwe Lumumba in September 2010—but she did not even know if she would be a match, since such a procedure would not be available in prison.[13]

That year, there were increasing actions both online, such as a "Day of Blogging" in March 2010,[14] and offline, including marches in Mississippi's capital, attended by many people, including prominent civil rights figures.[15] The case achieved increasing mainstream national awareness, including an editorial by the influential *New York Times* columnist Bob Herbert.[16]

The sisters have always maintained their innocence of the crime, though after a decade and a half of incarceration, guilt or innocence had come to seem less salient than questions about excessive sentencing. As one headline in late 2010 put it, "Sisters May or May Not Be Guilty, but Mississippi Assuredly Is."[17]

SUSPENDED SENTENCES, ON CONDITION: KIDNEY DONATION FROM ONE SISTER TO THE OTHER

The sought-after pardon was not to come. Mississippi governor Barbour instead declared that their sentences should be "indefinitely suspended," on the condition that Gladys donate a kidney to Jamie. In Barbour's statement on the suspension of their sentences, he noted:

> Jamie Scott requires regular dialysis, and her sister has offered to donate one of her kidneys to her. The Mississippi Department of Corrections believes the sisters no longer pose a threat to society. Their incarceration is no longer necessary for public safety or rehabilitation, and Jamie Scott's medical condition creates a substantial cost to the State of Mississippi.[18]

He also laid out the peculiar condition of Gladys's release:

> Gladys Scott's release is conditioned on her donating one of her kidneys to her sister, a procedure which should be scheduled with urgency.

In this statement on their release, there is neither acknowledgment of excessive sentencing nor compassion for a gravely ill woman. Yet since

Barbour was a contender for the Republican presidential nomination at the time, many analysts suggested that the release reflected his desire to appear racially tolerant and compassionate for national audiences.[19] At the same time, as an article in the *American Journal of Bioethics* pointed out, "by suspending their sentence on medical grounds instead of pardoning them outright, Barbour can remain 'tough on crime' while acquiescing to the sisters' supporters and saving the state about $200,000 per year in dialysis costs."[20]

It is worth unpacking the two reasons that Barbour gave for suspending the sisters' sentences: that they were no longer a threat to society and that releasing them would save the Mississippi taxpayers money. The first is striking for its "no longer"—it strains credibility to suggest that the sisters, who have never been accused of any crime except for involvement in this one robbery, were ever a serious threat to society. Barbour's rhetorical move erases the long-standing injustice with a temporal framing. The second reason is more obviously insidious and part of a broader neoliberal logic of governance: Barbour has explicitly and repeatedly said that he was interested in saving the taxpayers of Mississippi the money that the prison system was paying for Jamie Scott's expensive dialysis treatment.

In January 2011, Jamie and Gladys Scott were finally released, after serving sixteen years.[21] The sisters' release was long overdue and worth celebrating, a testament to the activism around the case. And yet the fact that the sisters were not simply pardoned makes for an incomplete victory.

Barbour's executive orders for the release of the Scott sisters were explicit that "the indefinite suspension of sentence" "may be revoked at any time, without notice or hearing, for violation of any condition set out by the Mississippi Department of Corrections or for any reason deemed sufficient by the Governor at his sole discretion."[22] Even aside from the extraordinary condition of organ donation in this case, suspended sentences allow only a very limited form of freedom. The sisters' unpardoned felony convictions effectively exclude them from the labor force as well as the right to vote.[23] They must pay for the administration of their parole, some fifty-two dollars a month, and so their freedom is literally not free.[24] They have endured police harassment since their release, occasioning the editorial comment in Jackson's African American newspaper that "nothing is free for the Scott Sisters; not even the Florida highway."[25] The year following their conditional release, in Barbour's final days in office, he pardoned an extraordinary number of prisoners, but the Scott sisters were not among them.[26]

Neither the sister-to-sister transplant nor the reincarceration has come to pass. In the months after their release, reports emerged that the sisters were too unhealthy and obese to be eligible to give or receive a kidney.[27] Years of health and logistical challenges followed: Jamie was making progress after weight loss surgery but lost a foot to amputation, and the expense of staying in a hotel to remain near the transplant center for follow-up care after surgery was onerous.[28] Gladys turned out not to qualify as a donor, and although Jamie eventually received a transplant in 2019, it was not from Gladys.[29] Their parole continues, yet there are no signs that they are being returned to prison. Nevertheless, this narrative of prison release conditional upon organ donation is a revealing site for considering how incarceration plays a role in the constitution of racialized biological citizenship in the United States.

MASS INCARCERATION AND ACCESS
TO CITIZENSHIP AND HEALTH

No other country has an incarceration rate as high as that of the United States, and our prison system is rooted in our history of slavery.[30] I refer to the U.S. prison system as "our" prison system, at the risk of sounding parochial to non-U.S. readers, to underscore the responsibility that I and others writing from this critical location must take for this moral emergency. At the end of the nineteenth century, in the wake of the fall of Reconstruction after the U.S. Civil War, the swelling prison system in the South did more than appropriate labor; incarceration and a prison record also became a mode of denying citizenship rights more broadly.[31] The Scott sisters have themselves put their experience into this larger context of the social role of criminal justice in perpetuating racial inequality. For example, the sisters participated in a town hall meeting at a Jackson church on the topic "Saving Black Boys from the Cradle to Prison Pipeline to Help Ourselves."[32] And speaking via Skype at a forum in Brooklyn, Jamie Scott herself said, "When I was a little girl . . . my grandma used to tell me . . . slavery is not dead in the south, it's called the law now."[33]

Barbour's notion of prison release as a way of saving money points to the peculiar character of the right to health care in the United States. As sociologist Anthony Ryan Hatch has pointed out, in the United States, the only people with a constitutional right to health care are prisoners; [34] any state is perfectly within the law to disregard the health of any ordinary citizen. This peculiar structuring of the right to health care—such that deprivation of liberty and access to a right to health care are explicitly intertwined—is part of how citizenship is negotiated in the United States, by institutional actors such as states and diverse health care providers as well as by people.

The U.S. Supreme Court has ruled that failure to provide adequate medical care to prisoners is considered "cruel and unusual punishment" under the Eighth Amendment to the U.S. Constitution. Thus Mississippi is not legally allowed to disregard the health of a person in its custody in prison. In the 1976 ruling *Estelle v. Gamble,* the Supreme Court liberally cites a still-active provision of the Civil Rights Act of 1871, which provides federal recourse for those whose constitutional rights are being violated by a state.[35] The Supreme Court's invocation of a Reconstruction-era law hints at the state and federal racial politics at stake in requiring states to provide health care for their prisoners.

By making the state's release of the Scott sisters conditional upon the state's release from any obligation toward them at all, a perverse form of freedom is constituted. Mississippi officials have explicitly articulated medical release of prisoners as a means of shifting costs from state to federal obligation.[36] If released prisoners qualify for Medicaid, a program for poor and disabled people jointly funded by states and the federal government, Mississippi's financial burden for their care is lowered to 25 percent. If released prisoners qualify for Medicare, a national program for Americans over the age of sixty-five, the financial burden is completely shifted to the federal government. And in this particular case, the sisters were allowed to move to Florida, where their mother, children, and grandchildren were living. The permission to move across state lines is an unusual privilege for people on parole, and while it is morally just and compassionate, that move also effectively diminishes still further any contribution by the state of Mississippi to their care. Any Medicaid or other state contribution for the Scott sisters' care will be paid for by the state of Florida, not by the state of Mississippi.

The Scott sisters case is embedded within the larger problematic of the public health consequences of mass incarceration.[37] As early as 1991, as the prison population was starting to grow tremendously, the American Public Health Association issued a statement decrying mass imprisonment on the grounds that "prisons disproportionately confine sick people . . . and . . . prisoners are subject to further morbidity and mortality in these institutions," noting that this burden falls particularly heavily on poor people and people of color.[38] Now that more than two million people are in U.S. prisons at any given time—by far the highest number and highest rate in the world—the racially disparate impact of incarceration not only on prisoners but also on their families and communities is widely recognized in public health scholarship.[39]

More recently, amid scholarship showing that Black/white health disparities are smaller among prison populations than among the general population, Dumont and colleagues point out that much of the impact on the social determinants of health appears after prisoners are released, creating "a perverse relationship between public health and incarceration: even as correctional facilities appear to provide a venue for addressing health disparities by accessing a high-need, medically-underserved, largely non-White population, incarceration itself ultimately perpetuates those disparities in the community."[40] Any health gains of African American prisoners from prison's access to care are undone postrelease. As authors in the medical journal *The Lancet* point out, "although current incarceration has mixed effects on prisoners' health, past incarceration has a clearly deleterious impact on health."[41]

Of course, even though prison confers a right to health care, in practice, prisoners are often very poorly cared for. That Jamie Scott was in such poor health—after spending essentially her whole adult life in the custody of the prison—points to the inadequacy of that care. The living conditions of incarceration, including poor nutrition, which play a role in health problems like Jamie Scott's, are foundational to the bodily control that the flawed medical care in prisons extends.[42] Dialysis itself provokes comparisons with incarceration—it is routine for nonincarcerated people with end-stage renal disease to describe themselves as "doing time."[43] In this sense, Jamie Scott's kidney failure is its own life sentence. Even the kidney transplant does not free her from the obligations of disease management but trades one intensive medical regime for another, albeit a less onerous one. And the medical system that cared so poorly for Jamie also demanded bodily sacrifice from Gladys.

The structurally racist criminal justice system is the context of both Jamie's organ failure and Gladys's offered donation, in a way that resonates with analyses of organ donation in low- and middle-income countries. For example, in her account of dialysis and kidney donation in Egypt, Sherine Hamdy posits that "disease processes" of kidney failure and survival are "already political" along lines of class and access to welfare services and "contest the very opposition between the biological and the political."[44] Both Jamie Scott's organ failure and Gladys Scott's promise of organ donation are rooted in their racialized class position and relationship to the state and thus have what Hamdy would flag as a "political etiology."

After their release, the sisters cared for their ailing mother (since deceased), while striving to get themselves healthy enough for transplant surgery, for which they lacked the necessary financial resources.[45] They eventually crowdsourced the funds. The inadequacy of health care for prisoners is in this sense continuous with the inadequacy of health care for racially stratified American publics.

BIOLOGICAL CITIZENSHIP IN THE U.S. CONTEXT

Many readers will have heard of legal scholar Michelle Alexander's highly influential book *The New Jim Crow: Mass Incarceration in an Age of Color Blindness*. That book persuasively argues that the denial of full citizenship that was explicitly racialized in the early twentieth century as "Jim Crow" was renewed in a putatively color-blind way through the intensification of mass incarceration, especially through the War on Drugs that has been pursued in a way that differentially exposes Black and poor communities to the criminal justice system and in turn differentially denies citizenship rights.

Here, I extend this engagement with citizenship rights to consider what scholars in the sociology and anthropology of biomedicine have termed "biological citizenship." I describe how this term emerges from two related literatures: one developed for analysis of resource-poor settings and the other for rich countries. I argue that oppressed populations within the United States can be betwixt and between, enrolled in both kinds of biological citizenship projects. The Scott sisters' extraordinary experience at the intersection of organ donation and incarceration can provide valuable insight into biological citizenship in the United States.

The first way of thinking about biological citizenship emerges from scholarship of postsocialist contexts, especially from anthropologist Adriana Petryna. Petryna has given a rich account of fieldwork in post-Chernobyl Ukraine, "where an emergent democracy is yoked to a harsh market transition, the damaged biology of a population has become the grounds for social membership and the basis for staking citizenship claims."[46] Petryna defines biological citizenship as "a massive demand for but selective access to a form of social welfare based on medical, scientific, and legal criteria that both acknowledge biological injury and compensate for it."[47]

The second way of thinking about biological citizenship emerges from scholarship of contexts characterized by consumer capitalism and advanced biomedicine and has been developed by sociologist Nikolas Rose and his colleagues. They make an explicit contrast with post-Soviet contexts in which demands are being made of the state and argue that the most relevant biological citizenship projects in "the West" are less nationally oriented and are "taking place within a 'regime of the self' as a prudent yet enterprising individual, actively shaping his or her life course through acts of choice."[48]

To understand the U.S. context, both deprivation and expressive choice are at stake—and the Scott sisters case can help to tease out how.

First, how might we think about the contours of American biological citizenship in Petryna's terms—negotiations over scarce state recognition and medical resources that invoke medical, legal, and scientific criteria to stake out membership in the U.S. body politic? Petryna's form of biological citizenship is being negotiated when prisoners demand the right to health care and is being both validated and denied when prisoners are released because of illness: release from prison somewhat restores the citizenship of the ill prisoner, but it also releases the state from obligation.

Indeed, a key contrast between the United States and "the West" in general is that the United States lacks a guarantee of baseline material security or access to health care. This leads to a resonance with biological citizenship forms in resource-poor settings, such as the "therapeutic citizenship" that Vinh-Kim Nguyen describes in West Africa. Nguyen writes about contexts of participation in HIV drug research and activism for drug access "in a setting where the disease may be the only way to get any of the material security one usually associates with citizenship."[49] He compellingly argues that therapeutic citizenship has "emerged as a rallying point for transnational activism in a neoliberal world in which illness claims carry more weight than those based on poverty, injustice, or structural violence."[50] Yet it matters that Nguyen draws his contrasts between West Africa and Canada, rather than between West Africa and the United States, because the United States is an exception to what he characterizes as the norm in rich countries.[51] The situation of incarcerated and formerly incarcerated people in the United States is like the West African one in that "widespread poverty means that neither kinship nor a hollowed-out state can offer guarantees against the vicissitudes of life."[52] Nguyen describes therapeutic citizenship as particularly "thin" compared to places with stronger states, where both Rose's and Petryna's biological citizenships are enacted.[53] Yet the biological citizenship rights of the Scott sisters are by no means thick. For the Scott sisters, as in Nguyen's site, "profoundly ethical predicaments shaped the therapeutic citizenship that emerged in places where other forms of citizenship could not be relied upon to secure life itself."[54] Illness claims by the poor can carry more weight than social justice claims "here," too, most blatantly in the case of the incarcerated. Leaving "the West" uninterrogated renders invisible the radically uneven thickness of biological citizenship within the United States.

Prison activism as a site of antiracist politics should itself be understood as a biological citizenship project. Experiences of imprisonment informed the health activism of the Black Panther Party,[55] and in her analysis of that political movement, Alondra Nelson calls for "a return to the work of Adriana Petryna and, in particular, to the milieu of catastrophe and deprivation that impelled her theorization of biological citizenship."[56]

Some analysts have suggested that, indeed, Rose's prudential and expressive model of biological citizenship does not apply in contexts of deprivation.[57] But even in a landscape of mass incarceration and profound deprivation, I would suggest that the "first world" model captures something important about the transformative power of biological knowledge, and it is why Gladys's offer to donate a kidney to Jamie should not be understood in terms of coercion but acknowledged to be an expressive act in which transplant medicine becomes a site of kinship and care as well as entrepreneurial choice. Participation in donation, of blood or of organs, is part of participation in biosociety in these terms. For example, as Jessica Martucci has argued, young gay male would-be blood donors' contestation of the Red Cross exclusion of men who have sex with men from its donor pool "has less to do with the national blood supply, and everything to do with access to a political forum in which citizenship claims can be made and listened to."[58] Michele Goodwin, a legal theorist of organ donation who is attentive to the experiences of African Americans, argues that the quasi-ownership of the body by both a potential organ donor and the donor's kin is "one way of looking at rights connected with the power to donate."[59] It is not clear at the outset which presents a deeper denial of prisoners' independent personhood: denying a "right" to donate and receive organs in an act of kinship and care[60] or demanding organ donation in exchange for release.

We might also note that Gladys's offer to donate a kidney to her sister should be understood as authentically expressive of her Christian commitments, in a way that is distinct from "the West" in general but characteristic of the United States. The valorization of organ donation in the United States draws on two distinct conceptions of eternal life: a consumerist fantasy that the body can be forever fortified[61] and the Christian veneration of giving of one's body that another might live.[62] In the United States, and especially in Mississippi, Christianity is not just a past that informs the present but a living site of the pursuit of succor and justice. The Black church has been an important site of advocacy for the Scott sisters, as it has been for prisoners in general. This articulation travels well throughout U.S. society.[63] Throughout the West, organ donation is framed by a broadly Christian trope: a demonstration of the laudable characteristic of altruism—the "gift of life"—and so the fact that Gladys Scott is willing to give her kidney to her sister demonstrates that she is a good person and may fortify public sympathy even among those who lack compassion for those unjustly imprisoned.

At stake here in antiprison activism as it intersects with the right to donate and receive an organ transplant is not any essential idea of *race* but a contestation of *racism*. Any ontological anxieties about the reality of race are beside the point, and race is not operating as a site of eugenic control. Indeed, in the Scott sisters' case, any genetic notions play an expressive role rather than a eugenic one: their genetic tie naturalizes the specific plausibility of kidney donation from one sister to the other. Notably, this is very different from the role that genetics usually plays in the analysis of race and racism in biomedicine. In this case, genetic ties become the site of kinship and care among individuals, rather than, as many critics of race in contemporary biomedicine contend, being the means by which specious notions of essential biological differences between members of different racial groups are reinforced.[64] And yet the expressive elements of biological citizenship in this case are inextricable from the mobilization of biological suffering to make demands for scarce resources. As anthropologist of race and biopolitics Jonathan Xavier Inda has explored in his work on race and pharmaceuticals, calling attention to the experience of bodily suffering of African Americans can become a locus of solidarity.[65] Mass incarceration and its contestation are vital sites for this project.

I argue that these models of biological citizenship and of therapeutic citizenship should be combined to understand the biopolitics around the Scott sisters case and the role of mass incarceration in constituting biological citizenship in the United States more broadly. The United States is simultaneously a society of scarcity and deprivation negotiated through biological diagnoses and legal categories, and of expressive agency enacted in biological terms, and of struggle for life amid abandonment by the state. Indeed, the tensions between racialized exclusions, the promise of consumerist freedom, and the lack of expectations of the state are foundational to a distinctly American biological citizenship.

Notions of biological citizenship that elide distinctions between and within rich countries evacuate their particular racial histories; the United States was founded on racial genocide and racial slavery as fundamentally as it was founded on notions of liberal democracy, and race remains fundamental to the new biocitizen, as it was to the old.[66] Moreover, the new biological citizenship does not simply replace the old. Any understanding of biological citizenship in the United States should not ignore the radically unequal access to biomedical consumption in America and the role of racialized incarceration in structuring access to health care and exclusion from personhood.

If we are to grapple with biopolitics in the United States, both our famously high-tech medicine and our infamously unequal access to it are fundamental. Our very bodies are shaped by our historical and contemporary contexts, characterized by both radical disenfranchisement and rhetorics of just treatment. In the United States, prison is not just a metaphor for power and control but a major way of organizing bodies in space and of constituting and depriving citizenship. Free at last, the Scott sisters and their supporters won a significant victory as they negotiated this terrain. The inhumane conditions imposed on these sisters by the state are a grotesque instantiation of disparities in access to citizenship and health, but one that reflects a broader context.

PRISON AND THE BODY IN THE CONTEXT OF MASS INCARCERATION

Barbour's perverse condition is extraordinary but not unprecedented. In 2007, state legislators in South Carolina considered a bill that would have shortened, by 180 days, the sentences of prisoners who agreed to donate a kidney. As legal scholars have pointed out, this represents a collision of two markets: the open market of criminal justice plea bargaining and the closed market of human body parts.[67] Plea bargains for reduced prison time are normalized forms of coercion, but the fact that prison power is enacted on prisoners' bodies becomes starkly explicit once the boundaries of the prisoner's body are called into question.

Although the South Carolina prisoner organ scheme was never enacted, it is not unheard of to exchange medical treatment for decreased sentences. Normally those are framed as crime prevention. The most prominent example of a quid pro quo of enduring medical treatment in exchange for release is so-called chemical castration for sex offenders.[68] Another example is anti-addiction pharmaceuticals for repeat drunk drivers, which sociologist Scott Vrecko has argued is perhaps emblematic of an emerging model, a shift from imprisonment to direct biological control.[69] The proposed South Carolina legislation and the Scott sisters case are different from these forms of control, because organ transplantation is not related to crime prevention. Chemical castration and anti-addiction pharmaceuticals are meant to prevent future criminal behavior, whereas the exchange of time for an organ highlights the ways in which prison sets up a debt relationship that is never closed.

In this sense, the transplant bargains are more of a piece with the routine character of criminal justice in the United States. Insofar as prison extracts a "debt to society" from the prisoner, the prisoner's body itself is always part of the payment. Extraction from the body in these cases points to an ever-demanding structure of debt peonage, analogous in a profound way to the debt peonage of the kidney sellers in India described by anthropologist Lawrence Cohen.[70] Debt constitutes the context for those in Cohen's account, which is a situation of poverty: "persons sell a kidney to get out of debt, but the conditions of indebtedness do not disappear."[71] Formerly incarcerated people in the United States are in a similarly fraught situation with regard to "debt to society," a debt that has theoretically been paid and yet is not erased. With suspended sentences, the continuation of the power of the debt is explicit. The sisters are in a situation in which both their financial sustainability and their legal freedom are precarious.

Moreover, also like kidney sellers in Cohen's account in India, incarcerated and formerly incarcerated donors in the United States face many bodily risks before and potentially from kidney extraction. Although the risk to the living donor is overwhelmingly described in abstract terms in bioethics literature, in an unequal world, risk is unevenly distributed. Living kidney donors from racialized populations in the United States on average have higher risks than white donors do: African American and Hispanic living donors have elevated risk of hypertension, diabetes, and chronic kidney disease.[72] In this case, Gladys Scott was less ailing than her sister but not healthy—indeed, although the full medical details are unknown, it seems that her own health was a reason that ultimately deemed her to be an inappropriate candidate as a donor.[73]

Paying attention to structural racism is also important for moving discussion of the Scott sisters case beyond a traditional bioethical approach, which would focus on whether it is ethical to offer Gladys Scott prison release in exchange for her kidney. In his discussion of the case, prominent bioethicist Arthur Caplan has put the focus precisely there, quoted on *ABC News* as saying "as soon as the governor began throwing around commutation—getting out of her prison sentence—he began to undercut the ethical framework."[74] Caplan's scholarly consideration of the issue is a bit broader and more grounded because it acknowledges both ethical concerns and practical issues that make organ donation by prisoners infeasible.[75] Yet there is no room in his framework for what Karla Holloway would highlight as "a cultural bioethics," how race and gender differentially constitute the independent personhood at stake in the Scott sisters' "private lives" that have become "public texts."[76] Neither is there space for reopening questions about the unjust treatment of the sisters before their conditional release or the ethics of mass incarceration itself. Indeed, interrogation of mass incarceration may present an opportunity for science and technology studies (STS) scholarship, as sociologists Laura Mamo and Jennifer R. Fishman have argued, to "participate in efforts that seek justice in ways that are associated with, yet distinct from, the study of ethics."[77]

Prison release in exchange for kidney donation does present an ethical problem, but we should resist putting it into a quandary paradigm, in which "a problem arises (what shall we do with the frozen embryos? shall euthanasia be authorized?) and ethicists spring into action."[78] As philosopher Anthony Appiah argues, ethical inquiry should not be so reduced. Anthropologist Paul Farmer, too, points out that posing questions as "ethical quandaries of the individual" dominates discussions of medical ethics, especially the decision whether to pull the plug on life support; in contrast, the everyday passively caused deaths of masses of poor people through denial of care are too rarely topics of ethical discussion.[79] Consideration of the Scott sisters case can exemplify this tendency, unless it is put into the context of the racialized system of mass incarceration.

This contextualization is resonant with recent scholarship of the ethical violations of the Tuskegee Syphilis Study[80] and brings to the fore different aspects of how medicine and structural racism are intertwined. Like the pervasive eugenically oriented and often deceptively implemented forced surgical sterilizations of Black women that the twentieth-century civil rights leader Fannie Lou Hamer evocatively decried as "Mississippi appendectomies" and coercive sterilizations of women prisoners that has continued well into the twentieth century, the coercive surgeries, in the Scott sisters case, justified on moral and cost-saving grounds, are consistent with rather than anomalies to broader social inequalities.[81]

From a biopolitical perspective, one of the things that prisons do is to instantiate exclusion from membership in the society whose life is fostered. In *Discipline and Punish,* Michel Foucault theorized that prison's obvious failure to rehabilitate is actually part of its function.[82] In the profoundly racialized U.S. prison system, the role of prisons in constituting a class of society that is excluded from society is particularly blatant.[83] Indeed, in the post–Jim Crow era, as sociologist Loïc Wacquant argues, the "carceral institution . . . has been elevated to the rank of the main machine for 'race making.'"[84] Wacquant argues that race-making institutions "do not simply process an ethnoracial division that would somehow exist outside of and independently from them. Rather, each produces (or co-produces) this division (anew)."[85] Prisons don't just reflect racial inequality; they are part of that inequality's construction.

The word *carceral* means simply "relating to a prison," and for Foucault, that extends well beyond prisons themselves to describe the broader systems of surveillance that control urban space. For example, systems ranging from surveillance cameras to electronic ankle monitors extend control well beyond the prison walls. The observation of the extensiveness of carcerality has been important in a growing body of critical race studies of science and technology, including by Ruha Benjamin, Nadine Ehlers and Shiloh Krupar, and Tony Hatch.[86] In this work, attention to control beyond the prison complements rather than replaces attention to the power of the actual prisons themselves. There is a danger in Foucauldian scholarship less attentive to race that the relationship of the term *carceral* to actual prisons becomes so abstract as to become almost metaphorical—but in the United States, both surveillance deploying carceral logics and prisons themselves contribute to the production of racial inequality.

The ethics of the event—the Scott sisters case—should not be extricated from an ethics of the uneventful: the routine structural violence of mass incarceration. Analysis of this case in these terms provides an opportunity to consider not only the residue of a horrific history and the specter of an unacceptable future but also the unbearable present.

4

Environmental Racism

PROTECTING GM'S MACHINES WHILE
ABANDONING FLINT'S PEOPLE

In April 2014, the city of Flint, Michigan, changed municipal water providers from the Detroit Water and Sewage Department, that had supplied it with water since 1967, to a new enterprise called the Karegnondi Water Authority, which planned to build a new pipeline to the same source: Lake Huron. This was a shady deal in many ways, entered into by an unelected emergency financial manager, that placed all of the financial risk of building the new pipeline onto the heavily indebted city. While that pipeline was being built, the city would switch to using water from the Flint River.

Almost immediately, Flint's human residents complained about the look and smell of the water from the new source, but these complaints were dismissed and ignored by city managers for years.

Representatives of the most prominent corporate resident of Flint — the car company General Motors — complained about the water quickly too: within the first few months, they noticed that the new water supply was corroding the machinery at their Flint engine plant.[1] In October 2014, the GM plant reached an agreement with a nearby township to buy water from the old water supplier and switched its source.[2]

Flint's human population of 102,000 residents would not start getting any relief whatsoever for another year after the GM plant switched back. By that time, thousands of the city's children had been exposed to demonstrably brain-damaging levels of lead.[3] In January 2016, Michigan governor Rick Snyder and U.S. president Barack Obama declared a state of emergency, mobilizing Michigan National Guard troops to distribute bottled water and Federal Emergency Management Agency funds.[4] The water source for the people was finally switched back in October 2015. But the root of the problem was not the toxicity of the water in the Flint River but rather that the water was corrosive to metal, and so it drew toxic metals out of the pipes in which it was being transported.[5] Thus, by that time, these pipelines were already so corroded by inadequately treated water from the Flint River that any water that subsequently flowed through them remained toxic.[6] Some of the pipes have finally been replaced such that some homes now have access to safe water, and some of the children have started to receive compensatory educational services, but the crisis for human health is still ongoing.[7]

In this chapter, I argue that the differential protection of the material integrity of GM's machines over the bodily integrity of the people of Flint provides a window into racialized biopolitics. I frame the contrasts between the machines that were protected and the pipes and humans that were disregarded in terms of access to citizenship: who can make successful claims—especially but not only against the state—for access to safe water and, with it, material and bodily integrity? The chapter follows such disparate nonhuman objects as fiscal bonds, machines, and pipes to track the intertwined flows of capital, labor, and water, in order to illuminate crucial stratification *within* both human and nonhuman categories. In Flint, the city's creditors and GM's machines received quick care, while the vulnerabilities of the pipes and the population were initially disregarded. The protection of finance and machines over pipes and people illustrates the devaluation of groups of humans considered to be surplus in the service of the interests of capital. This small event within the broader Flint water crisis illustrates a fundamental element of racial disparities in health in the United States: differential protection of financial capital and racialized human life. To contest environmental racism, we need a more-than-human politics that critically centers those people who have been framed as being outside of "the society that must be defended."[8] Infrastructures and environments do connect us all, but paying attention to how they do so in ways that are stratified is an essential part of understanding how they shape contemporary inequalities in citizenship and health.

FLINT AND GENERAL MOTORS

As with each of the twenty-first-century cases explored in this book, the preferential treatment of GM's machines over Flint's people emerges out of a much longer history. General Motors was founded in Flint in 1908, and the journeys of the company and of the city have been deeply intertwined. This history, in turn, has also been one about race.

The jobs offered by companies like General Motors were among those that catalyzed the "Great Migration" of African Americans from the southern states. In 1910, 90 percent of African Americans lived in southern states; by the end of the Great Migration, in 1970, 47 percent of African Americans lived outside the South.[9] Of course, industrialization drew many groups to cities like Flint, including white immigrants. When the city's population peaked at two hundred thousand in 1960, Flint was majority white. However, like most deindustrializing cities in the United States, Flint has experienced "white flight," in which the white population of cities migrates out disproportionately—archetypally to the suburbs, but also beyond, including to rural areas and to other states. As of the 2010 census, the population had declined by half and was 56.6 percent Black.[10]

Before its water crisis, Flint was brought to mainstream attention beyond the borders of Michigan by Michael Moore's breakout film *Roger and Me,* in which the city is figured as an emblematic site of corporate abandonment and deindustrialization.[11] In that 1989 film, Moore pursues the CEO of General Motors, Roger Smith, to confront him about the closure of several auto plants in Flint. Despite record profits, GM had decided to move a great deal of production to Mexico to lower labor costs. Flint's organized workers had reached the middle class by the late 1970s, when eighty thousand people were employed at GM plants there. This broad-based prosperity emerged out of a long labor history: the Flint Sit-Down Strike of 1936–37 was a foundational event of the United Auto Workers labor union.[12] The film attends to the tremendous impact the 1980s plant closures had on the city of Flint. GM's disinvestment in Flint continued after *Roger and Me*: there are now just eight thousand people working at GM plants in the area; that is, compared with its peak, 90 percent of the car-manufacturing jobs in Flint are gone. Even as GM remains a dominant force in Flint—politically, economically, culturally—the extent of the company's abandonment of the city and its people is profound.

RACIALIZED EMERGENCY MANAGEMENT

The fateful 2014 change in water source was made under the authority of an unelected political leadership: emergency managers appointed by the state governor to impose fiscal austerity on the city. Since 1988, the state of Michigan has passed a series of legislation that allows the state to take control of local governments that are in financial distress—defined as failing to pay their payroll or debts. The laws allow the state government to replace local elected officials with emergency financial managers selected by and answerable to the governor.

The mechanism of emergency financial management has allowed a state government dominated by white Republicans to take over Black-majority school systems and Black-majority cities.[13] The eight cities that have been put under emergency management are home to less than 10 percent of the total population of Michigan, but they are home to half of the Black population of Michigan.[14] This makes the power of emergency management in Michigan starkly resonant with colonialism in the sense of the practice of taking control over another country or territory. In that familiar model, colonial authorities might make promises to improve the conditions of local populations through ordered management, but the political structure overwhelmingly serves the ends of economic exploitation by the colonizers.[15]

In the wake of the Flint water crisis, some commentators dismissed the claim that racism played a role by pointing out that one of the two emergency managers who signed off on the fateful decision to switch water sources is African American.[16] But this ignores a fundamental question of the location of political power: whose interests was that person appointed to serve? The selection of Black emergency managers is part of the neocolonial emergency management process, not an exception to it.[17]

The subversion of democratic processes facilitated by "emergency management" imposed by the state of Michigan was a key source of the water crisis. In theory, the emergency managers could be imagined to be the ones responsible for looking out for the people of Flint. They were, after all, appointed to replace the elected officials with that charge. For complicated reasons to which I will return, it is the case that the people of Flint were suffering under onerous water bills, some of the highest in the country. There is an absurdity even to that baseline situation: an economically struggling population in the middle of a state surrounded by fresh water was paying more than those living elsewhere in the state, in other major cities, or in desert cities like Phoenix. But rather than providing the population with relief from their burdens, the emergency managers exacerbated their suffering.

The emergency managers had a far narrower task than looking out for the people of Flint: they were responsible for looking out for the *finances* of Flint. Even this they arguably did not do, as they favored a risky investment in a new water source that has certainly not turned out to be financially sound. There was the promise of eventual cost savings with the new water provider, though the risks were high enough and the savings marginal enough that it's not clear why the state was so enthusiastic about the switch.[18] Yes, Flint residents' high water bills precrisis put them in a position of high rates of delinquency, which was part of the justification for the emergency need to change to a water supplier who would charge lower rates. But there were other, far less risky ways of addressing the problems of high water bills faced by residents if the emergency managers had truly had the needs of residents as their top priority.[19] Instead, city managers saw an opportunity to invest public capital in a new pipeline and took it.[20] The difficulty that residents had in paying their water bills did not seem to be the motivation for the change—and in the wake of the crisis, Flint residents have faced tax liens and foreclosures on their homes over unpaid water bills, while the city's debt to the Karegnondi Water Authority continues to accrue.[21]

Indeed, there is something even more fundamental at stake here that has particular relevance for those interested in health: in Flint's economic model, with its high unemployment, care for city finances does not align with care for the city's pipes or population. "Care" here is a question not of affect or feeling but of practical work undertaken in an emergent situation.[22] The emergency managers' disregard for Flint's people contrasts with the care that GM took for its machines: the company's care for corporate finances does align with looking out for the well-being of its corporate assets—its machines. In a city and economy characterized by abandonment, the machines have value for their owners that ensures their care. In the process, public finances become extricated from investment in public goods—infrastructure for the population—and servicing private actors takes precedence.

Emergency managers were empowered to break almost any contracts—including with, for example, unions and pensioners—but *not* empowered to break contracts with bond holders.[23] That is, obligations to citizens were subject to renegotiation, but obligations to financial institutions were nonnegotiable—even agreements signed during the scourge of pernicious banking practices that would lead to the financial crisis of 2007. Moreover, the emergency managers had the authority to enter into new contracts with bond holders. As such, the provision of funding for a new pipeline to be built by a new water authority was treated with extraordinary urgency, whereas the provision of safe water to the people of Flint was not.

In the discursive frame of emergency management, the city of Flint is denigrated as a fiscally irresponsible individual, while the abandonment that caused its financial duress is obscured.[24] Honoring obligations to pensioners and unions is framed as "financial irresponsibility" while honoring obligations to banks is framed as "financial responsibility"—a technocratic ideology that only pretends not to be ideological.[25] As activist Claire McClinton points out in the ACLU documentary *Here's to Flint,* "it's interesting to note, in Public Act 436, the Emergency Manager cannot void a contract with bond holders. That's off limits. Bond holders are sacred. They cannot be touched. People are not sacred."[26] Even in the wake of the crisis, during which time Flint has signed a contract to stay with the Detroit water supplier for thirty years (now reorganized after its own bankruptcy process and called the Great Lakes Water Authority), the city remains liable for the debts to which its emergency managers agreed in order to build the pipeline from which it now never plans to draw water.[27]

Decisions about when more debt is tolerable and when it isn't are always political decisions—something that came to the fore frequently in national U.S. politics during the Obama administration, for example, in the sovereign debt crisis provoked by congressional Republicans in an effort to repeal Obamacare.[28] There is a parallel here with structural adjustment in poor countries: state spending on health is a common target for austerity measures, whereas taking on debt for infrastructure projects of dubious value provokes fewer questions from financial sectors. In Flint, assuming an onerous bond to pay for a new pipeline was presented as debt that the city of Flint could afford, while maintaining the status quo or seeking a better deal with the existing water provider was presented as unsustainable.[29] From a financial perspective, one might say that debt is figured as sustainable if it is capable of generating a return—and managers were operating on the assumption that investing in the people of Flint cannot generate a return, whereas investing in a pipeline can.

WHY ARE GM'S MACHINES AHEAD OF PEOPLE IN THE LINE FOR SAFE WATER?

The conditions of poverty and dispossession in which the people of Flint found themselves prior to the water crisis, and the inaction in the face of need during the crisis, both exemplify *institutionalized racism,* as outlined by epidemiologist Camara Jones. For Jones, "institutionalized racism" manifests in both "material conditions" and "access to power."[30] Relevant aspects of *material conditions* in this case include disparate access to "sound housing" and "a clean environment." The role of *unequal access to power* is exhibited in the unchecked actions of the emergency manager. In a wealthier, whiter city, those seeking to profit from water provision would not have had the ability to disregard citizens' concerns so completely.[31] Finally, what Jones characterizes as "inaction in the face of need" was fundamental both to the baseline situation and to the management of the crisis.[32] While there is an identifiable perpetrator (the emergency manager), as in many instances of institutionalized racism, he is not an isolated villain but an element of much larger structures of dispossession.

The roots of emergency management lay in the same late-1980s economic conditions underlying *Roger and Me*: an economic structure of massive unemployment for the population, while the owners of capital continued to prosper. Racial capitalism in Flint epitomizes a politics of abandonment: no longer figured as surplus labor "reserve" for capital, the people of Flint are figured as incapable of contributing anything to wealth accumulation and so are abandoned by capital and the state.[33]

There are resonances between the emergency management approach used in Flint and structural adjustment policies imposed on postcolonial countries by global financial institutions in the wake of World War II and especially since the 1980s.[34] Structural adjustment policies require that countries follow neoliberal policies of "free markets" over social services. They move fundamental decisions about economic priorities out of the local sphere and onto outside organizations—the World Bank and International Monetary Fund in the case of postcolonial countries, the emergency managers appointed by the state in Michigan's deindustrializing cities.

In this context, the ability of GM to intervene on behalf of its machines shows that the market is not simply "free." Not just any company owner can call the governor of Michigan and make a successful plea for the protection of the company's machines. But GM plays an especially important role in Michigan, historically and today. This is not to say that GM always looks out for its machines—it has abandoned plenty, sold off others for a pittance. Yet machines can be and often are figured as ahead of humans in the line for resources. In the classic anticapitalist short film *Island of Flowers,* pigs are ahead of ragpickers in the line for organic waste repurposed as food, because pigs have an owner who has money, whereas the impoverished people in this part of Porto Alegre, Brazil, have neither an owner nor money.[35] The people of Flint might once have been "owned" by GM—initially in a sense of "wage slavery" that, because of union organizing, gave way to better working conditions even as a profound power imbalance continued between capital and labor—but the company no longer needs them and so no longer lays claim to them. But the company does look out for its machines.

GM can even make a claim that looking out for machines is looking out for humans—the eight thousand remaining jobs, the economy of the city and the state on which many more humans rely. But this is perverse. The experiences of those in Flint reveal that the increasing shift from human labor to machines is not the techno-utopia that it pretends to be. Although automation is supposed to render only human labor obsolete, rather than the human itself obsolete, the perceived value of people of color and of their labor is never fully extricable in the logics of capitalism — and obsolescence follows racialized lines.[36] Automation is often argued to enhance human safety: rather than humans doing the hard and dangerous labor, machines would do it, and so the humans' bodily integrity would be protected. But exclusion from labor does not lead to bodily safety, because racialized bodies rendered economically surplus are also bodies rendered disposable.

It could conceivably have been the case that the damage to the engines at the GM engine plant would have acted as a red flag, providing evidence that the worries that the people of Flint had about the new water were well grounded.[37] However, that is not what happened: the knowledge generated by the corrosion of the machines did not translate into actionable knowledge to be applied to the humans. The machine corrosion was addressed promptly, while the flesh corrosion that was continuous with a long history of violence against racialized populations remained unseen — or, perhaps more precisely, denied or dissembled.[38] The machines were protected, while the humans were met with inaction in the face of need.

There might be something evocative about the detail that the most dangerous impact of the toxic water is on humans under construction (i.e., children) and cars still under construction (both the preassembled parts and the machines that assemble them). But children and machines need water differently. How might we reorder the prioritization of their needs?

WATER'S CITIZENSHIP RELATIONS

Water is a vital part of our material and social world, and attending to its quality and distribution offers a distinctive entry point for consideration of access to citizenship and health. For feminist theorists interested in "thinking with water," water's fluid nature provides an opportunity to consider the interconnectedness of two very different imaginations of "currency"—flows of capital and of the seas[39]—and water should be understood as *relation* rather than *resource*.[40] Engaging and extending this scholarship, I am interested in what forms of citizenship relations we can see in the preference for machines over people in the Flint water crisis.

When President Obama addressed the people of Flint, he framed access to safe water as a basic right of citizenship: "I will not rest . . . until every drop of water that flows to your homes is safe to drink, and safe to cook with, and safe to bathe in, because that's part of the basic responsibility of a government in the United States of America."[41] The specificity of the patriotism mattered: as many observers noted, the people of Flint were relegated to treatment "like a third world country." GM's machines, however, maintained full U.S. citizenship.

Indeed, the privileging of privately owned nonliving machines in Flint is emblematic of political recognition in the context of late capitalism. In the United States, corporations are legally treated as "persons," and, as legal theorists Marc de Leeuw and Sonja van Wichelen argue, our period is characterized as "a time when legal personhood is dominated by global capital, one where corporate personhood is profiting more from naturalized forms of legal personality than any human being is able to do."[42] Do the natural human persons resident in Flint have the standing to make human rights or citizenship claims?

Because water is essential, people have to pay whatever is charged for it, and if only toxic water is on tap, that's what they have to buy. Of the five hundred largest water systems in the United States, Flint charged its residents the highest rates, and residents were not in a position to demand either affordability or quality.[43] GM is large and powerful enough that it can negotiate rates—or seek out an alternative supplier—but individual people cannot. In a narrow technical sense, GM's switch to the previous water provider was possible because the GM plant was adjacent to another township (a spatialization that is itself the product of a complicated history of corporate strategy of suburbanization of manufacturing).[44] However, similarly positioned individuals would not be able to make that kind of choice on their own. Moreover, if individuals are not able to have their collective interests advocated for because their governments can't or won't negotiate on their behalf, they are trapped.

We might understand the differential treatment of GM's machines and Flint's humans as illustrative of differential "hydraulic citizenship," in the terms of anthropologist Nikhil Anand. In his ethnographic account of the water infrastructure in Mumbai, Anand argues that "the ability of residents to be recognized by city agencies through legitimate water services is an intermittent, partial, and multiply constituted social and material process."[45] In Flint, we can see that GM has a privileged form of citizenship relative to the population and can extend that privilege to machines that it owns.

In suggesting that GM has a privileged form of citizenship, I am specifi-cally *not* referring to what has become known as "corporate citizenship." This is a neoliberal trope of "corporate social responsibility" that praises small, environmentally sound or community-minded endeavors, often as a means of concealing more fundamental exploitation.[46] In contrast, the form of citizenship that I am talking about is the form that can make demands for services from government. There is something obscene about the fact that while GM claims to be a good citizen of Flint, when it came to the emerging Flint water crisis, it used its citizenship rights only to claim resources for itself, not to be a good neighbor to those who are supposedly fellow citizens.

One of the central insights of science and technology studies (STS) is that power is not located in human relations alone but in a complex network of relationships among human and nonhuman actors. This has been part of the growing appeal of STS, as more academic fields become interested in the "nonhuman," "posthuman," and "more-than-human." As long as stratification among humans is not ignored amid the analyti-cal elevation of these other domains, this move has a great deal to reveal about contemporary biopolitics.

ENDURING INEQUITIES IN MORE-THAN-HUMAN POLITICS

Foregrounding the role of water in fostering the material and bodily integrity of nonhumans who share our environments can be invoked to mobilize a sense of common cause between humans and other organisms. In STS, much interest in the nonhuman looks to the organic: animals, most prominently, but also bacteria, plants, and nonorganismic forms of life grown in laboratories. One of the impulses that this scholarship often foregrounds is common cause between human and nonhuman life, in the face of deadly capital. Looking out for nonhuman organisms is not essentially discontinuous with looking out for ourselves as human organisms. However, it certainly can be discontinuous, if care for non-human life comes at the expense of consideration of the stratification of environmental racism.

As anthropologists have argued, contestation over whether water is a natural resource, a right of citizenship, or a market good is a characteristic of the neoliberal context of many parts of the world.[47] The cruel conditions that the people of Flint have faced raise this question: should water be treated as a right of citizenship, rather than as a market good? Or perhaps the stakes are even more fundamental: should access to water be a human right? Posthumanist feminists have urged a move beyond a "human right" to water, because of its anthropocentrism: all life depends on water, not just human life.[48] This would suggest that nonhumans, too, have some form of citizenship rights—but how to square that with the fact that not all humans have such rights fulfilled?

Importantly, because it is often rooted in explicitly intersectional feminism, a great deal of posthumanist feminist scholarship foregrounds the racial stratification among humans produced through these processes of capital accumulation and the distribution of toxic water. For example, feminist historian and technoscience scholar Michelle Murphy's work on a place not far from Flint—the nearby waterway of the St. Clair river—highlights the impact of pollution on both Indigenous people and fish.[49] There is occasionally a somewhat mystical quality to her mode of story-telling, as it locates the chemical industry spills of the past as shaping the human and nonhuman reproductive potentials of the future. In the bigness of the story, and especially the timeline, the unbearable present of chemical violence and its racialized impacts risks receding from focus.[50]

Thinking with water is most useful if we pay attention to the profound unevenness of its flows, in Flint and beyond. Doing so has the potential to contribute to another intertwined strain of scholarship attentive to the nonhuman: one that looks to infrastructure. The most celebrated example is Jane Bennett, whose book on "vibrant matter" includes a chapter on the failure of the electrical grid on the East Coast of the United States.[51] One might analyze the Flint water crisis itself as a failure of infrastructure; it was the infrastructure itself that poisoned the water of Flint. As I noted at the start of the chapter, the issue was not a toxic water source but inadequately treated water that drew the toxic metals out of the pipes in which it was being transported.[52] And in the face of that infrastructural failure, humans and nonhumans were in some sense brought together: we often think of machinery as less vulnerable than humans, but both are subject to the corrosive impacts of water—and bottled water is an even more implausible alternative for a manufacturing plant. However, the differential protection of GM machines versus human Flint residents shows how the infrastructure's failure is not universal but instead stratified.

Any critique of anthropocentrism that loses sight of the most marginalized in society risks creating an abstraction that ignores the way in which capital itself gives a preferential option to the machines, as long as those machines have owners and generate returns. Hierarchies follow lines not only of non/human bifurcation but also of ownership and, with it, obsolescence.

CONTESTING SLOW VIOLENCE: FLINT LIVES MATTER

Tellingly, Flint activists hearkened to Black Lives Matter to lay claim to the mattering of their own lives with the slogan "Flint Lives Matter."[53] Even as the slogan is mobilized by a multiracial coalition of activists, it is importantly distinct from the insidious right-wing response to Black Lives Matter that seeks to minimize the centrality of racism in the organization of protection of bodily integrity with the claim that "All Lives Matter." It is a racialized process of dispossession that has rendered Flint lives disposable—from General Motor's disinvestment to the state's imposition of emergency financial management—and this is highlighted rather than obscured in Flint Lives Matter activism.

The concept of the "preferential option for the poor"—an idea drawn from Catholic liberation theology that has also been influential in medical anthropology[54]—is useful for understanding the power of both the demand that "Black Lives Matter" and the overlapping demand that "Flint Lives Matter." Standing with and advocating for the most marginalized in society is both worthy on its own terms and a vital part of advocacy of the common good.[55] This kind of commitment can seem a bit old-fashioned amid the posthumanist turn, on one hand, and the attention to climate on a global scale, on the other, but the Flint water crisis can illuminate the ongoing salience and even urgency of specificity.

A great deal of environmentalist activism emphasizes the shared burdens of environmental risk: we are all in this together, in that we all live in the same environment. There is a problematic potential for environmental activism to contribute to the All Lives Matter evasion, rendering the vulnerability of Black lives even more analytically marginalized by bringing flattened imaginaries of "humanity" or even "life" to the center of the scope. Both posthuman scholarship and environmental activism should analytically foreground those who are structurally most vulnerable to environmental harms. Yes, we are all connected through infrastructures and environments. However, they connect us in ways that are stratified and stratifying and recognizing this interplay is vital to understand how they shape contemporary inequalities in citizenship and health.

The Flint water crisis broadly and the ability of GM to shift water sources while the people continued to suffer offer an unusual opportunity to explore through the lens of an event the kind of environmental racism that usually operates slowly and insidiously. Most environmental racism operates in a way that is unspectacular—what Rob Nixon has called "slow violence":

> By slow violence I mean a violence that occurs gradually and out of sight, a violence of delayed destruction that is dispersed across time and space, an attritional violence that is typically not viewed as violence at all. Violence is customarily conceived as an event or action that is immediate in time, explosive and spectacular in space, and as erupting into instant sensational visibility. We need, I believe, to engage a different kind of violence, a violence that is neither spectacular nor instantaneous, but rather incremental and accretive, its calamitous repercussions playing out across a range of temporal scales.[56]

As Nixon highlights, the slowness and relative invisibility of these kinds of harms pose challenges for contestation. Flash points like the Flint water crisis provide an opportunity for contestation insofar as they are instantiations of, rather than exceptions to, slow violence.

In Flint, as with all of the cases in this book, the ethics of the event should not be separated from the ethics of the uneventful. As we saw in the chapter on the spike in chronic disease in the aftermath of Hurricane Katrina, urban infrastructure and its failure are sites of biopolitics, in which the lack of protection of Black lives constitutes societal exclusions. Even in a terrain of more-than-human politics, stratification among humans in relationship to capital and political power is fundamental. Demands for access to safe water are inextricable from demands for social and political inclusion—indeed, they point to the urgent necessity of the dismantling of institutionalized racism.

5

Police Brutality

ENFORCING SEGREGATION AT A POOL PARTY

In June 2015, fifteen-year-old Dajerria Becton was among the African American teenagers at a pool party in the Dallas suburb of McKinney, Texas, who were violently suppressed by the police. The incident was captured on cell phone videos that were widely disseminated, which included a powerful image of the small bikini-clad girl's bodily vulnerability under the knee of a police officer. Close attention to the McKinney incident—both the violent policing of the suburban pool itself and the dissemination of the viral video—provides a window into how racism and antiracism are renewed and refigured in the twenty-first century.

This chapter is a bit of an outlier in the book as a whole, because it is the one least directly related to health, as generally defined in fields such as medical sociology—this event did not take place in a health care setting, and it did not cause an acute instance of illness or death. And yet control of bodies in space, including through police violence, is interconnected with health. It is certainly *biopolitical.* As discussed in the book's introduction, in a biopolitics following from the French philosopher Michel Foucault, more is at stake than the state killing people—that has become rarer (albeit still all too common, especially in the United States). But the state is involved in setting up relations in which some bodies' flourishing is fostered and other bodies are relegated to conditions of suffering and death.[1] As quantitative sociologists have shown through analysis of zip code–level data, both segregation and intensive policing have tremendous impacts on health.[2] Differentially depriving Black bodies of access to recreational facilities and of the ability to move freely through space is part of the deprivation of flourishing. As many have become increasingly aware in this era of viral videos of police violence against Black people, police brutality is a source of acute injury and death. Even more pervasively, police brutality enforces segregation and stratifies well-being.

In this chapter, I take the opportunity to engage more directly with nonmedical technologies that foster and constrain bodily well-being. I will articulate and put into relation the plural technologies of race that come together in the McKinney encounter and its aftermath. As in the previous chapter on the Flint water crisis, some of these technologies are infrastructural elements of the built environments—here, recreational swimming pools rather than the pipes through which the water flows. The definition of technology includes but is not limited to the products of scientists and engineers, and it is inclusive of all of the tools with which humans shape and navigate our environments and which at the same time also shape us and constrain and facilitate our movements. I will attend to technologies that are lower tech, including swimsuits and police uniforms.[3] Particularly important here are media technologies— that is, technologies that both capture images and sound and distribute them—including cell phone cameras and social media. Surveillance is also fundamental to Foucauldian biopolitics, and the efforts to reverse the lens of observation have become a site of contemporary resistance.[4] At the end of the chapter, I connect the analysis of this case with media theorists' concepts of the "liberatory imagination" and "race as technology," to highlight not just constraints of racism but also creativity in antiracist response.

THE INCIDENT AND VIRAL VIDEO

It was a hot Friday afternoon in June 2015 in McKinney, Texas—a middle-class suburb of Dallas. Fifteen-year-old Dajerria Becton was among the African American teenagers celebrating the end of the school year at a pool party at the Craig Ranch neighborhood pool, a facility managed by the homeowners association. Multiple people called the police complaining about a disturbance there, but the nature of the disturbance was contested. Some called to report that uninvited teens were climbing over the pool's gate to access the already overcrowded space, defying the security guard.[5] One of the party's hosts described a very different originary flash point: Tatiana Jones, a nineteen-year-old African American woman who lived in the neighborhood and had invited classmates to enjoy a cookout outside the pool, described her guests being denigrated by two white women, who she recounted called her guests "black f-ers" and other slurs, and told her to "go back to [your] Section 8 home" and "go back where you're from," and who responded to Tatiana's defense of her younger guests by hitting her in the face, instigating a fight.[6] Tatiana and her mother also placed calls to the police, to report being attacked by these white women.[7]

Police response at the McKinney pool party was captured on a cell phone video by a white teen in attendance and was widely disseminated.[8] In the video, an enraged police officer named Eric Casebolt first chases down a group of Black teenage boys. Once he rounds them up and has them seated on the grass, he berates them: "Don't make me run around with fucking thirty pounds of goddamn gear on here in the sun, because you want to screw around out here." At a certain point he goes up to a group of girls that includes Becton and tells them, "Y'all keep standing here running your mouths, you're going to go, too." The girls initially talk back indistinctly but then start to disperse, Becton going a different direction from the rest. Inexplicably, the officer pursues her and pulls her down to the ground.

The images of the assault are distressing, and yet I include a pair of illustrative stills, because images will be focal objects of analysis in this chapter. In the video's most compelling moments, widely disseminated as still images online, the thin, dark-skinned teenage girl in an orange and yellow bikini is thrown to the ground by the white male police officer in uniform. In the video, we see Black boys rush over and shout at the officer in Becton's defense, and Casebolt points his gun at them to ward them off. Other people mill about. The officer pins Becton down and yells "on your face," kneeling on her back as he handcuffs her. Becton calls out for someone to call her momma and sobs under the weight of the officer's body.

The incident sparked outrage and protest, as well as compelling artistic responses to which I will return. It would become one among many viral

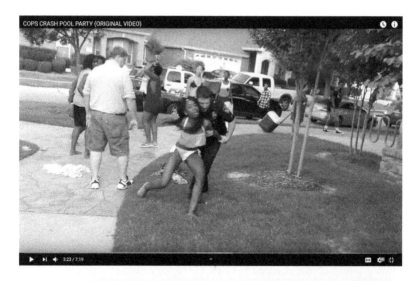

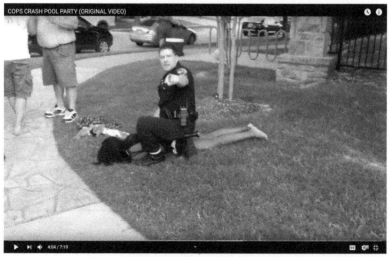

"Cops Crash Pool Party (Original Video)," cell phone video posted to YouTube by Brandon Brooks, June 6, 2016, https://www.youtube.com/watch?v=R46-XTqXkzE. The first still image shows a slight Black girl in a brightly colored bikini being pulled down from behind by a white male police officer. The second still image shows the girl lying face down on the grass and the white male uniformed police officer facing and pointing to the camera as he stoops over her with one knee on her back. Screen grabs by Katherine Behar.

videos of police violence that would catalyze the Black Lives Matter movement, which had been founded in 2013 after the acquittal of the vigilante
killer of Trayvon Martin in Florida and had grown with protests against
the 2014 police killing of Michael Brown in Ferguson, Missouri.[9] At the
McKinney pool party, there was no loss of life, and yet it is an evocative
case through which to explore the role of police violence in the enforcement of white supremacy and the urgent vitality of antiracist response.

THE SUBURBAN POOL AS A TECHNOLOGY
OF SEGREGATION

Segregation—the systematic separation of groups of people in space—
is a fundamental element of structural racism. Its operation generates a
terrain by which members of privileged groups have differential access to
coveted resources, ranging from well-funded schools to safe and comfortable leisure spaces. Police and vigilante violence, and even the threat of
it, is a mechanism by which racialized exclusion and control is enforced.

Swimming pools have functioned as sites of exclusion that are important both symbolically and literally. For social scientist of computing Jane
Margolis and colleagues, in their influential book *Stuck in the Shallow End:
Education, Race, and Computing,*[10] the lack of access to pools both leads to
an increased risk of drowning and operates as an analogy for lack of access
to computing. They argue that a violently enforced history of exclusion
has created a present situation in which Black children are assumed to be
"not interested" in or "not capable" of swimming and that these assumptions about Black lack of interest and capacity are also made with regard
to the white (and Asian) space of computer science.[11] Their focus is on
unequal access to the space to develop skills, because students of color
are more likely to have access only to basic computer skills at a young age,
but it's also worth noting that part of what is differentially lacking in both
swimming and computing is the space to *play*. Play is a vital part of how
young people learn to explore the world, and being excluded from play
spaces structures senses of belonging.

When public pools were introduced in the United States at the end
of the nineteenth century, they were austere places framed in terms of

"hygiene." They were meant to be places in which the urban poor of industrializing cities could access baths—and although sexes were segregated, races often were not.[12] By the 1950s, pools had transformed into the kinds of places that we recognize today, intended to promote "leisure," and had become the domain of white families—an exclusivity that the civil rights movement would contest.[13] If demands for access to pools were no longer framed as a health issue in the same way as they might have been in the hygiene era, the differential access to these pools and other spaces for physical activity has been and continues to be an element of differential access to both health-promoting physical exercise and simple fun.

Recreational spaces in general and pools in particular have long been central contested ground for segregation and resistance—and when African Americans successfully gained access to urban recreational facilities in the civil rights era in the second half of the twentieth century, whites largely abandoned them, and many public facilities closed or were privatized.[14] The white flight from the urban core in that period is an inextricable part of what spurred both the development of suburban communities like McKinney and the placement of homeowners association–controlled pools within them. The Craig Ranch neighborhood pool is a homeowners association pool and as such can be thought of as public only in a very restricted sense: it is for use by an exclusive public.[15] The contested distinction between public and private pools operates as a technology of race.

The racialization of the suburbs, especially in the South, has become more complex since the initial era of desegregation and white flight, and McKinney is an archetypal suburb of the New South. That is, its appeal does not necessarily draw on a backward-looking nostalgia for an antebellum South but on a forward-looking aspiration for an ascendant space of economic opportunity. McKinney had been named "best place to live" by *Money* magazine in 2014—with a median family income of $96,143 and a median home price of $217,879, with a combination of "Southern charm" and "growth-industry jobs" in defense and technology.[16] McKinney is overwhelmingly white—77.3 percent white, according to the U.S. Census Bureau, though that number decreases to 61.4 percent for "White alone, not Hispanic or Latino"; there is a significant minority "Black or African American alone" population of 11.5 percent.[17] These statistics are not too far off from the national averages, and that suggests the community has broad appeal. Yet segregation exists even in places like McKinney, which are far from the inner city and somewhat racially mixed: the newer, more upscale west side (in which this pool party took place) is much whiter and more prosperous than the older, less upscale east side.[18]

Segregation is precisely a reaction to the transgression of space.[19] It was Black affluence that motivated the intensification of segregation after the Civil War, on the trains and in so many other semipublic spaces that the small but emergent Black middle class might buy its way into.[20] The segregation of pools and the contestation thereof operates as a literal site of the enactment of racism.

The rules of the Craig Ranch neighborhood pool were that each member could bring in two guests.[21] Thus, the segregation being enforced is not total, but a racially loaded division between private and public still shapes the space. Although individual Black bodies of neighborhood members are allowed in the space, and even allowed to bring a limited number of guests, there is a tension underlying the inclusion that points to deeply engrained concerns that the space not be overrun. Assumptions about "who is and who is not 'from the neighbourhood'" are inextricably connected to racism.[22]

Ambiguity about whether people with the requisite amount of money could buy their way in spurred both suspicion as to whether Black people in middle-class spaces had indeed paid their way in and vigilantism and calls for authority control. This extends to the arguments that precipitated the McKinney incident, when white people at the pool hollered to "go back to Section 8 homes"—referring to a governmental rental assistance program that provides vouchers to low-income families to rent from private landlords, implying that the Black attendees must not be living there on equal terms with the white revelers. As sociologist Barbara Harris Combs has argued, the McKinney pool party incident is certainly part of a "Jim Crow State of Mind" in which Black "bodies out of place" are subjected to surveillance and violence.[23]

SEXUAL TERRORISM ENACTED BY THE MAN IN
THE POLICE UNIFORM AGAINST THE GIRL IN THE BIKINI

The racialized control of space in pools is inseparable from control of gendered space, and technologies of race are also technologies of gender. Until the turn of the twentieth century, pools were segregated by sex, but as pools increasingly allowed men, women, and children to swim together, there was a more prominent impetus for racial segregation—part of a broader panic over interracial intimacies and miscegenation.[24]

Swimsuits are blatantly technologies of gender, sorting and performing bodies that are on display, in ways that present normative bodies that are necessarily simultaneously gendered and racialized.[25] Even as the Miss America pageant has recently ended its swimsuit competition,[26] and "body-shaming" advertising featuring women in swimsuits has become increasingly marginalized,[27] the imposition and defiance of bans on burkinis in France underscores the stakes of swimsuits as sites of control over women's bodies.[28]

And yet bikinis can also be experienced as a site of fleeting freedom, as Black feminist historian of fashion Tanisha Ford highlights in her "Black Girl Song for Dajerria."[29] Ford describes Becton's suit as an "eye-catching" "multicolored neon bikini with a long fringe that hung from its top" and speculates about how Becton might have felt upon trying it on and deciding that it was "the one."[30] The suit would allow her to "stand out from the crowd," receive compliments from her friends, and even embody the affirmation "I *am* black girl magic."[31]

In the images at McKinney, we see the juxtaposition of the bikini and a radically different type of clothing: the police uniform, arguably a technology of racial terrorism insofar as it represents a key armed wing of the structurally racist state. Ford also highlights the contrast, arguing, "The very material restrictions and weight of the oppressive uniform against Casebolt's skin serves as a symbol of state violence. His words communicate a rage shrouded in envy of the black teens who frolicked around in more heat-appropriate attire, who dared to take pleasure in their own black leisure."[32]

Many Black feminists have put the McKinney incident into the context of sexual terrorism. How can we tell that the terrorism is both racial and sexual? One way is by considering what a different response there would have been if a Black police officer had pinned down a white teenage girl in this way—as Sikivu Hutchison has point out, "little black girls can never occupy the space of carefree, feminine innocence that little white girls expect as their birthright."[33] Black girls don't get the chance to be children. This is connected to one of the many elements that Ruth Nicole Brown, a leading voice in Black girl studies, describes as creating barriers to the freedom of Black girls: they are "routinely disciplined into taking up less and less space."[34]

The smallness of Becton's body calls our attention to the ways that racialized fantasies of Black dangerousness operate in police logics. What can explain the act of an officer throwing a child in a bathing suit on the ground? What can explain a grown police officer sitting on the body of a fifteen-year-old and publicly humiliating her? Helplessly on the ground and in a two-piece bathing suit, Becton screamed out for her mother as Officer Casebolt pulled on her braids and pushed his knee into her back. Becton herself attributed the response to the officer feeling disrespected by something that the girls said—as quoted in the *Guardian,* "He told me to keep walking and I kept walking and then I'm guessing he thought we were saying rude stuff to him," Becton told local news. "He grabbed me and he like twisted my arm on the back of my back and he shoved me in the grass, he started pulling the back of my braids and I was like telling him that he can get off me because my back was hurting really bad."[35] Nothing Becton might have said would have justified that response: as leading Black feminist cultural critic Brittney Cooper remarks in her essay about the event, "citizens have a right to 'mouth off' to the police."[36] And, as lawyer and Black Lives Matter organizer Nnennaya Amuchie points out, "barely 100 pounds, Becton presented no threat to Officer Casebolt, yet he grabbed Becton like a wild animal that needed to be tamed."[37]

Of course, it is also true that the threat perceived by police officers from unarmed Black men is rooted in fantasy. This was a particularly outrageous element of the self-justification for mortal force in the case of Michael Brown, in which the police officer justified shooting an unarmed teen at close range by describing the menace of his victim in animalistic or even superhuman terms.[38] Becton's treatment on that day in McKinney underscores the continuity between the experiences of Black boys and girls—although the majority of the attention to police brutality has focused on Black boys and men, Black girls and women experience disproportionate authoritarian control as well.[39]

MOBILIZING IMAGES OF POLICE BRUTALITY TO SPUR OUTRAGE AND DEMAND EQUALITY: THEN AND NOW

On a few levels, paying attention to the juxtaposition between the bodily vulnerability of Becton and the aggression of the police officer exemplifies historical continuities: swimming pools have been key sites of segregation in urban and suburban spaces, police have played an important role in enforcing that segregation, and images of police violence have been mobilized to galvanize resistance. At the same time, the images and their mobilization also reveal important elements specific to the twenty-first century.

Consider: here are images from the *New York Times* of a "swim-in" at a motel in St. Augustine, Florida, in 1964, in which both the hotel manager and a plain-clothes police officer intervened to enforce segregation—the manager pouring in toxic levels of acid cleaning fluid near the swimmers, the officer jumping in to physically disrupt the desegregated swim.

The heavy-handed police action against Black swimmers in private public space is in a sense a twentieth-century legacy that McKinney follows. In her classic essay "Race and/as Technology; or, How to Do Things with Race," to which I will return, media theorist Wendy Chun points out that "race has been so key to the definition of public and private as such."[40] That is, race undergirds the very constitution of both public spaces and private spaces and the idea of public and private as distinct and separate spheres. A key desegregating maneuver since the civil rights movement has been to hold private businesses to standards of public accommodations. Thus white supremacist responses have contested Black demands for inclusion in both public and private spaces, imposing barriers through rules and through vigilante and police violence.

Yet there are two key differences worth highlighting. First, the use of

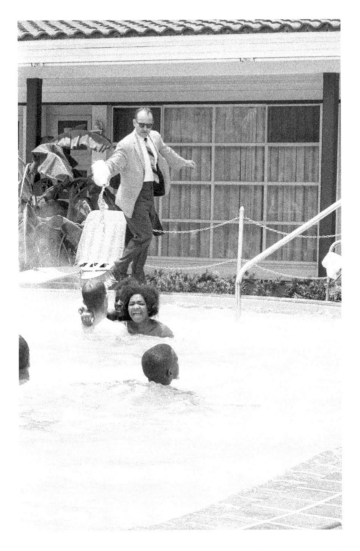

"James Brock Dumping Acid into Swimming Pool," June 18, 1964. In this iconic black-and-white photograph, a white male hotel manager in a jacket and tie, James Brock, pours acid from a large plastic jug into the pool of the Monson Motor Lodge in St. Augustine, Florida, to disrupt an integrated group of swimmers who are protesting the hotel's segregation policies. A few swimmers are visible in the foreground, including a white man and a Black man seen from behind, and another Black man whose face is partially obscured. At the center of the image facing the camera, a young Black woman named Mimi Jones is crying out. Photograph by Horace Cort, via Getty Images. Reprinted with permission.

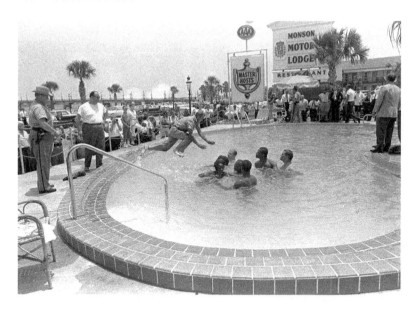

"Police Officer Jumps into Monson Pool to Break Up Swim-In," June 18, 1964. In this iconic black-and-white photograph, a fully clothed white man is jumping into the pool of the Monson Motor Lodge in St. Augustine, Florida, to disrupt a group of integrated swimmers—two white men, three Black men, and two Black women—who are gathered in the center of the pool. In the background, we can see onlookers, the motor lodge sign, parked cars, and palm trees. Photograph by Horace Cort/Shutterstock .com. Reprinted with permission.

cleaning fluid in the 1964 incident implies a biopolitical logic of hygiene and contamination that does not seem to be operating at McKinney. Second, whereas the "swim-in" was an organized protest that was professionally photographed by invited journalists, as was the norm in the civil rights era, the McKinney incident took place at an otherwise mundane end-of-year party, and the video was shot and distributed by a white teen who was a fellow pool party attendee. In the era of Black Lives Matter, how is visual media creation and distribution mobilized to interrupt contemporary racism?

During the civil rights era, activists together with their professional photographer allies contested and reconfigured public–private binaries as they demanded Black freedom to exist in and move through community spaces. Today, those mobilizing for racial justice by insisting that Black lives matter do so through the lenses of cell phone cameras—and through artists' pens.

ARTISTIC INTERVENTIONS TOWARD
A "LIBERATORY IMAGINATION"

Police officers (and their supporters) often justify the use of force by invoking the purported danger of the job, but with her slight build and exposed body, Becton obviously could not possibly have posed a physical threat to a police officer. This palpable absurdity became the subject of creative artistic response. Here, I turn to ways in which the cell phone video of the McKinney pool party incident was not merely distributed but also reimagined. Doing so builds on Ruha Benjamin's vital insight that "technology captivates" in multifaceted ways: capturing bodies on police cameras and crime prediction algorithms, capturing the imagination with regard to the allure of the technological fix, and also operating as a site for a more expansive "liberatory imagination."[41]

One critical take that circulated on mainstream media was a faux news report presented on the late-night comedy news program *The Daily*

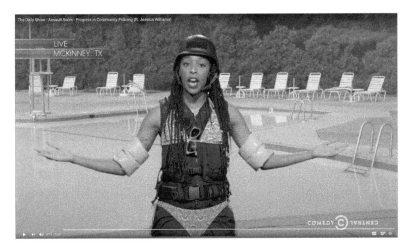

"Assault Swim," segment on *The Daily Show*, June 8, 2015. The image features Black female correspondent Jessica Williams in front of a deserted pool, wearing a bikini over body armor, a helmet, and swimming floaties. Screen grab by Katherine Behar.

Show, with correspondent Jessica Williams in full body armor and helmet accessorized with a pink bikini and blue floaties, which she referred to in the segment as a "McKinney Bikini."[42]

This six-minute segment titled "Assault Swim" featured a wide-ranging back-and-forth between the show's white host, Jon Stewart, and Black contributor Jessica Williams, referred to in the clip as the "Senior Texas Aquatics Correspondent." Host and correspondent discussed water guns—fun staples for white pool-party-goers, in a state in which white people famously carry real guns freely but Black people face mortal danger if suspected of having a gun. Stewart asks whether these kinds of police incidents are actually becoming more common or whether it only seems that way because of the presence of cell phone cameras. Williams responds, "I don't know, but either way, it's progress." She elaborates, "It's progress because the cop pulled a gun on a group of Black kids and nobody is dead."

In addition to the photographic images and video clips, the incident inspired captivating drawings. These kinds of images circulated widely online and often operated by illustrating the absurdity of the fantasy of racialized threat.

Consider this movie poster spoof that figures a Black teen in a bikini as the monster in a remake of *Attack of the 50 Foot Woman,* by Chicano syndicated cartoonist Lalo Alcaraz.[43] The giant girl does not really look like Becton, besides having long braids—both her skin and her swimsuit are lighter in shade, and her face is expressionless. She holds a police car with a flashing light in one hand as she stands, crouched and ready to attack, one foot up to her ankle in the pool and the other foot on the road. In the background, we see abstracted panicked white swimmers, pool chairs, a fence, and rows of cookie-cutter houses. There are three pieces of text: a small "McKinney Texas Police Productions presents" at the top, the headline "Attack of the 14 Yr. Old Black Girl" in the top left corner, and the pseudo-threat "No cop is safe!"

This cartoon resonates with another compelling drawn inversion of positions, by Markus Prime, that was featured in *Teen Vogue.*[44] In that cartoon, a Black female figure in an orange bikini stands with her foot on a subdued and handcuffed white male uniformed police officer—the girl's

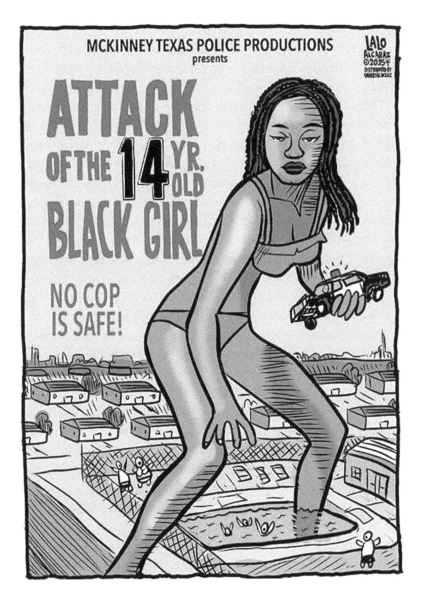

Lalo Alcaraz, *Coming Soon: Attack of the 14-Yr.-Old Black Girl!,* June 10, 2015. A cartoon in the style of the movie poster for *Attack of the 50-Foot Woman,* in which a giant Black girl in a pink bikini has one foot in a swimming pool and a police car in one hand. Suburban houses in the background are dwarfed in size by the giant Black girl. LA CUCARACHA copyright 2015 Lalo Alcaraz. Distributed by Andrews McMeel Syndication. Reprinted with permission. All rights reserved.

stance like that of a successful trophy hunter or conqueror. The color of the girl's skin and bikini are more similar to Becton's, and yet in this cartoon, too, the image is not literalistic: both the girl and the police officer are drawn without faces, figured as archetype rather than representation.

These kinds of images operate as a commentary on contemporary racism and illustrate that race is being done a bit differently in an era of cellphone video–enabled social media than it was in the civil rights era. Unlike the 1964 St. Augustine swim-in, the McKinney pool party video was shot not by a professional journalist serving as an invited witness of activists but by a (white) teen who happened to be at the same pool party. Whereas the iconic images of the civil rights era are organized of events that were professionally mediated by observers who were purportedly "objective" yet obviously sympathetic, the McKinney images, like many iconic images of the Black Lives Matter era, have been unplanned and mediated by amateurs who are openly taking sides with the victims. The materiality of the images is different, in ways that matter for how the injustices that they depict are framed and disseminated: the swim-in photograph needed to be developed and printed before it could be distributed along well-defined media channels; the digital video of the McKinney pool party incident was ready for immediate upload and nearly immediate, widely dispersed distribution. Even as a few voices within the mainstream media—notably on the right-wing Fox News network—resisted seeing the humanity of the victims and sided with the police even after being confronted with the damning video,[45] broadcast and print media broadly followed the narrative as it was structured by the amateurs.

It's worth noting that in many of these artistic reimaginations of the McKinney pool party incident, an abstracted Black girl is represented, rather than Becton as a recognizable individual. In civil rights–era depictions, we don't for example just see a Black woman sitting on a bus; Rosa Parks is always specifically Rosa Parks. Abstraction makes it more possible to imagine different Black girls in the same situation, and this generative layering of the concrete and the imaginative is a strategic tool in the era of Black Lives Matter. The use of less recognizable images here captures something of a tension between #SayHerName, which underscores the individual identities of Black women who have suffered violence, especially at the hands of the police, and the politically powerful extrapolation that frames specific violence as simultaneously a broader condition of Black women's experience even for those whose names are not known.[46] As communication scholar Sherri Williams observes, "#SayHerName forces people to recognize the humanity of Black women victims of violence"[47]—a recognition of humanity that is not circumscribed but rather strives to encompass and extend.

Communication technologies are important here but are not somehow inherently on the side of justice. As communication studies scholar Armond R. Towns argues, "#SayHerName operates as a Black geography because it both relies on and contradicts Western modes of communication. It is a digital usage of the master's tools to challenge 'his' supremacy, but feminists like Audre Lorde might question whether such a challenge is indeed effective."[48] Because technology is designed by and for elites, inequality and injustice cannot be solved simply with technology. Yet the creativity itself is worth appreciating, and to embrace technology as a tool of resistance is not necessarily to buy in to a fantasy of a technological fix.[49]

Whereas some have argued that increasing the ubiquity of cameras will somehow automatically decrease racially disparate policing,[50] we should be skeptical. Indeed, technologies presumed to be less biased than people have often operated to intensify inequalities, in what Ruha Benjamin has termed the "New Jim Code," an "insidious combination of coded bias and imagined objectivity" in which "innovation . . . enables social containment while appearing fairer than discriminatory practices of a previous era." A riff on Michelle Alexander's *The New Jim Crow,* which argues that mass incarceration has allowed the continuation of racial segregation and discrimination in purportedly color-blind form, the New Jim Code "considers how the reproduction of racist forms of social control in successive institutional forms (slavery, Jim Crow, ghettoization, mass incarceration), now entails a crucial sociotechnical component that hides not only the nature of domination, but allows it to penetrate every facet of social life."[51]

The noninnocent quality of technology is one reason why, for those who advocate for justice, art becomes a vital complement to technology. The deprofessionalization of video representations of racism-in-action is importantly extended as the images are appropriated, reinterpreted, and reinvented in irreverent ways. These irreverent moves are, I think, of a piece with what Ruha Benjamin points to in her call for "abolitionist tools" for the New Jim Code—inverting the hegemonic logics by which technology reinforces long-standing racial hierarchies. Benjamin points out that these antiracist interventions are often in the realm of the speculative or the fictional, and indeed, it is revealing that it is not just the cell phone camera footage itself but also the speculative inversions in the artistic interventions inspired by it that seem to capture something important about both the world in which we live and the world as we would have it be.

THE CONSTRAINT AND CREATIVITY IN "RACE AS TECHNOLOGY"

This foregrounding of media brings in opportunities to analyze race in new ways, informed by media theorists such as Beth Coleman and Wendy Hui Kyong Chun, who have explored how race can be understood as a technology rather than as a natural fact.[52] As Chun argues, the idea of "'race as technology' shifts the focus from the *what* of race to the *how* of race, from *knowing* race to *doing* race by emphasizing the similarities between race and technology."[53] The kinds of creative interventions that emerged in response to the McKinney pool party incident focus attention on race as technology—that is, not on ontological questions about what race *is* but on more procedural questions of what race *does*.

Chun uses the phrase "race and/as technology" to highlight the insepa-rability of being and doing, and both authors foreground how technological infrastructures are a constitutive part of racialization. The opportunities that this approach offers come later in Chun's piece: "race as technology is both the imposition of a grid of control and a lived social reality in which kinship with technology can be embraced."[54] Within science and technology studies, this approach has been more common among those who study media and information technologies rather than those who study biomedicine. Media theorists of race tend to be more open to the generative potential of technology than to biomedical theorists of race, yet contemporary biopolitics needs this attention to technologies as well, especially as the analysis moves beyond explicitly medical spaces.

Considering race as technology reframes what it means to articulate or contest the reality of race, such that the stakes are not about essences but about actions within a system of constraints that have real-world impacts. As Coleman explains, "the claim of race as a technology recognizes racialized identities as constructed—understanding that, within the construct, if you die, you really are dead. If one is caught on the wrong side of the law with the wrong color or accent, then it may be curtains, lights out. That is the 'reality effect' of race."[55] That is, Coleman embraces the now-conventional idea in humanities and social sciences that "race is socially constructed" but wants to put the emphasis on what that construct does in the world and how we navigate it. It's striking that Coleman draws on a term from literary theory—the Barthesian "reality effect"—to describe how the constructed notion of race has material effects. Importantly, it points to a particular sensibility in which there exists a potential for reinvention, for repurposing the tools of race for another world that might be possible.

If we understand racial inequality as fundamental to the simultaneously material and imaginative world in which we find ourselves, we should see ourselves as both characters and authors. Coleman argues that "race as technology also grasps a prosthetic logic in which local agency—yours and mine—depends on what we make of the tools at hand."[56] In this pool party incident and in the artist and activist response, the tools at hand include suburban swimming pools and cell phone videos, white police bodies wielding handcuffs, and Black teen bodies in bikinis. The existing structures are powerful, such that communities almost always stay segregated and exposed Black bodies are almost always vulnerable—and yet artists and activists point to the potential for alternative realities.

The technologies that came together in this incident are both involved in the imposition of control and involved in technologically mediated activist and artistic tactics that seek to intervene on that social order. This is true of the making and the dissemination of the video itself, which is a mode by which a white boy can take some modicum of action in the face of police violence against his Black friends, and it is true of the wide-ranging artistic responses.

It is important not to overstate the transformative nature of amateur videos of police violence, but it is worth attending to how the videos do things with race that both build on the role of professional journalistic photography in the civil rights era and reconfigure visual media production and dissemination for differently participatory pathways. The channels through which these videos circulate, including but not limited to YouTube, do not have the same kind of gatekeeping as does mainstream media, and they allow a kind of peer-to-peer sharing that can be useful for activism.[57] Insofar as videos like this provide mobilizing resources for Black Lives Matter, they offer potential tools for making race do different things: illuminating operations of power precisely to resist and subvert them and to affirm the humanity of Black people in the face of a dehumanizing society. Coleman elaborates with a suggestion of what race might do otherwise: "in asking the reader to consider race as technology, I also participate in the critique of racial instrumentalization, but in a fashion that exploits the nature of technology toward the human and the affective as opposed to toward dehumanization."[58]

I'd like to conclude by drawing on one final point from Chun that is useful for scholars of racism and health. She writes that understanding race and/as technology "displaces ontological questions of race—debates over what race really is and is not, focused on separating ideology from truth—with ethical questions: what relations does race set up?"[59] Scholars of race and biomedicine in science and technology studies are still overwhelmingly engaged in the debunking move—adjudicating what race is and is not—with the notable exception of those who work at the intersections of biomedicine and Afrofuturism, such as Ruha Benjamin and especially Alondra Nelson.[60] Broadly, scholars of media are much further along in considering race and/as technology than are scholars of health and medicine, and these analytical domains and approaches should be more fruitfully brought together to understand how bodily well-being is stratified in a structurally racist society. Attending to technologies does not distract from the human stories here but elaborates them. Whereas so much of the scholarship of racism and health focuses on how technologies divert our attention from fundamental inequalities,[61] we can see in this case that technologies can foreground rather than obscure human experiences. Indeed, technologies ranging from swimming pools to video-sharing platforms are inseparable from human experience and as such are vital sites for understanding both the constitution of race and the contestation of racism.

6

Reproductive Injustice

SERENA WILLIAMS'S BIRTH STORY

On September 1, 2017, tennis star Serena Williams gave birth to her daughter Olympia.[1] As is all too common for Black women in the United States, the event was life threatening. Her experience reveals the inadequacy of frequent explanations for high maternal mortality among Black women, such as poverty or failure to seek prenatal care. Even with all of the resources, expertise, and assertiveness that she was able to muster, Williams faced challenges in receiving the attention and intervention that she desperately needed. This chapter puts Williams's account of her experience into the context of two intersecting elements: connections between Williams's birth experience and those of far too many Black women and representations of Williams's body over the course of her career that have combined hypervisibility with dehumanization. Doing so highlights the ways in which Black women's bodies are simultaneously hypersurveilled and inadequately cared for. As a star within a neoliberal sports context, Williams is not an uncomplicated advocate for justice for Black women, yet there is rich potential for reproductive justice advocacy as she mobilizes her social media platform to call attention to racial disparities in access to safe births and to demand change.

Serena Williams is by any measure a major star. Not only is she a premier tennis player—a former world number 1 many times over with more major singles titles than anyone else (male or female) since the establishment of the professional tennis circuit in 1968—she is also a crossover celebrity, with huge endorsement deals, and she is extensively discussed in mainstream media and on social media. As a muscular and expressive Black woman who has often not conformed with the specific white feminine ideals of the sport in terms of either physique or behavior, she has been the subject of a very high degree of scrutiny. And yet in her experience of childbirth, she faced perilous invisibility.

A HARROWING EXPERIENCE

In an interview-based account published in the fashion magazine *Vogue,* Williams tells readers that she had an easy pregnancy, but dangerous fetal heartbeat changes during labor led to an emergency surgical delivery by Cesarean section (C-section).[2] Baby and mom were both fine at that point, but the next day, Williams had shortness of breath that, because of her history with blood clots, she immediately recognized as a pulmonary embolism. According to the *Vogue* article, "she walked out of the hospital room so that her mother wouldn't worry and told the nearest nurse, between gasps, that she needed a CT scan with contrast IV and heparin (a blood thinner) right away. The nurse thought that her pain medication might be making her confused. But Serena insisted, and soon enough a doctor was performing an ultrasound on her legs."[3] Serena reflected, "I was like, Doppler? I told you, I need a CT scan and a heparin drip." Serena described the experience of struggling to get the right test in an HBO Sports documentary, her voice trembling with emotion: "I'm like, listen, I need you to run a CAT scan, with dye, because I have a pulmonary embolism in my lungs, I know it—I've had this before, I know my body."[4] Once the medical staff finally did proceed to give her the CT scan, the blood clots settling in her lungs were confirmed, and she was given the drip that she needed. She said, "I was like, listen to Dr. Williams!" Several days of surgical medical interventions followed, to deal with Williams's postpartum complications.

Williams made the story public in a Facebook post that featured a cute video of her baby daughter with this commentary:

> I didn't expect that sharing our family's story of Olympia's birth and all of complications after giving birth would start such an outpouring of discussion from women—especially black women—who have faced similar complications and women whose problems go unaddressed.

These aren't just stories: according to the CDC, (Centers for Disease Control) black women are over 3 times more likely than White women to die from pregnancy- or childbirth-related causes. We have a lot of work to do as a nation and I hope my story can inspire a conversation that gets us to close this gap.

Let me be clear: EVERY mother, regardless of race, or background deserves to have a healthy pregnancy and childbirth. I personally want all women of all colors to have the best experience they can have. My personal experience was not great but it was MY experience and I'm happy it happened to me. It made me stronger and it made me appreciate women—both women with and without kids—even more. We are powerful!!!

I want to thank all of you who have opened up through online comments and other platforms to tell your story. I encourage you to continue to tell those stories. This helps. We can help others. Our voices are our power.[5]

For Serena Williams, it was a choice to align her story with the cause of addressing Black women's high maternal mortality.[6] As an unquestionably extraordinary woman who made it through the ordeal in the end, she might well have seen her experience as a singular one and moved on. She chose instead to articulate her experience as part of Black women's experience. This is not to say that she denied her privilege relative to other Black women. In a subsequent interview published in the magazine *Glamour,* she underscored the unfairness of the fact that many women in her situation would not have been listened to, even after insisting, and, referring to the mortality statistic in her Facebook post, said, "If I wasn't who I am, it could have been me."[7] As she has increasingly done in recent years, she took advantage of her high-profile platform and direct access to audiences online to raise awareness about this important social justice issue.[8] A Black woman shouldn't have to be a superstar to survive.[9]

Williams's advocacy in her Facebook post—especially her insistence that "EVERY mother deserves a healthy pregnancy and childbirth" and her appreciation of all women, whether or not they have children—resonates with the Black feminist–led social movement called *reproductive justice.* Reproductive justice centers a broader understanding of freedom

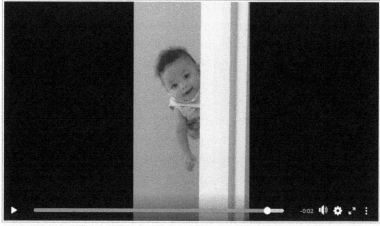

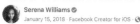

Serena Williams ✓
January 15, 2018 · Facebook Creator for iOS · 🌐

I didn't expect that sharing our family's story of Olympia's birth and all of complications after giving birth would start such an outpouring of discussion from women — especially black women — who have faced similar complications and women whose problems go unaddressed.

These aren't just stories: according to the CDC, (Center for Disease Control) black women are over 3 times more likely than White women to die from pregnancy- or childbirth-related causes. We have a lot of work to do as a nation and I hope my story can inspire a conversation that gets us to close this gap.

Let me be clear: EVERY mother, regardless of race, or background deserves to have a healthy pregnancy and childbirth. I personally want all women of all colors to have the best experience they can have. My personal experience was not great but it was MY experience and I'm happy it happened to me. It made me stronger and it made me appreciate women -- both women with and without kids -- even more. We are powerful!!!

I want to thank all of you who have opened up through online comments and other platforms to tell your story. I encourage you to continue to tell those stories. This helps. We can help others. Our voices are our power.

👍❤️😮 27K   1.6K Comments 1.4K Shares 843K Views

 Share

Image from a Facebook video by Serena Williams in which her baby, Alexis Olympia Ohanian Jr., is looking around a corner, with accompanying text describing her surprise at the level of response to her sharing the complications she experienced during childbirth, referencing statistics about racial disparities in maternal mortality, voicing support for all women, and urging more women to share their stories. Below, we see that 27K people have reacted to the post, with "like," "love," and "wow," and it has received 1.6K comments, 1.4K shares, and 843K views. Facebook post by Serena Williams. Screen grab by Katherine Behar.

than "reproductive rights" generally does.[10] Whereas reproductive rights generally focuses on access to contraception and especially abortion, reproductive justice not only demands access to these vital means to prevent pregnancy and birth but also demands the transformation of broader social conditions to enable safe birth and parenting. This is a necessary intervention, because as influential Black feminist legal scholar Dorothy Roberts highlights, access to abortion or lack thereof is not the only impediment to reproductive liberty that Black women face in a country that has long sought to decrease Black birthrates, including through forced sterilizations and involuntary forms of birth control.[11] This history in turn informs the work of SisterSong Women of Color Reproductive Justice Collective, which "defines Reproductive Justice as the human right to maintain personal bodily autonomy, have children, not have children, and parent the children we have in safe and sustainable communities."[12] Community seems to be part of what Williams is reaching for in her post. And her words also resonate with the demand made by SisterSong and reproductive justice advocates more broadly: "Trust Black Women."[13]

The relevance of Serena Williams's birth story for reproductive justice was underscored for me at an event at Georgia Tech in Atlanta in March 2018: Dialogue on Race, Biomedicine, and Reproductive Justice, cosponsored by the Working Group on Race and Racism in Contemporary Biomedicine and the Black Feminist Think Tank.[14] The Dialogue featured one of the founders of the reproductive justice movement, Loretta Ross, in dialogue with public health scholar Whitney Robinson.[15] In the Q&A portion of the event, one questioner identified herself as a student at Spelman—a renowned historically Black women's college also located in Atlanta—who wanted to become a gynecological oncologist. Saying that she believed that Black women's increased mortality was due to their fear of the medical system and waiting too long to go to the doctor, the student asked, how can medical professionals encourage Black women to seek preventative care and not just treatment? Loretta Ross's response was to question the assumptions underlying the student's framing, pointing to the experience of Serena Williams in childbirth. Even with all of the fame, power, status, and name recognition that she had, Williams was still not believed by her health care provider. One of the other members of the audience chimed in, saying, "And talk about someone who is in tune with her body!" And yet, Loretta Ross reminded us, Williams almost died, as too many Black women do. Ross encouraged those of us gathered at the event to focus "upstream," on the untrusting health care providers.

The call to shift the focus from patient distrust to provider distrust resonates with anthropologist Dána-Ain Davis's work on "reproductive injustice." Davis argues that rather than blaming Black women for their own poor health outcomes, health care providers "must look racism in the face and question the ways that the system within which they work might contribute to racist outcomes, draw from racist discourse, or perpetuate racist ideas."[16]

Sociologist and writer Tressie McMillan Cottom mentions the post-childbirth interview with Serena Williams in her essay on her own tragic birth story: "In the interview, Serena describes how she had to bring to bear the full force of her authority as a global superstar to convince a nurse that she needed treatment. The treatment likely saved Serena's life. Many black women are not so lucky."[17] McMillan Cottom had been trying to get medical attention for pain and bleeding during pregnancy, but her concerns were dismissed. After giving birth to a preterm baby who died soon after her first breath, McMillan Cottom was chided by health care workers: "you should have said something." But she *had* spoken up; the problem was that, as a Black woman, she had been "presumed incompetent."[18]

Any individual woman might have difficulty being listened to by her health care provider, and indeed the medical complaints of women in general are all too often dismissed.[19] Yet the magnitude of the inequality makes it clear that there is a racialized pattern when it comes to experiences in childbirth. As Williams notes in her post, racial disparities in maternal mortality are stark: indeed, according to the CDC, in the United States "pregnancy-related mortality ratios are 3–4 times higher among black than white women."[20] The causes of Black women's high risk of morbidity and mortality in childbirth are highly contested. As with so many health disparities, the question of race is sometimes reduced to socioeconomic class—and with it, education and access to care. And yet the maternal health and infant mortality disparities are so great that middle-class Black women with college degrees have worse outcomes than poorer white women with less than a high school education.[21]

Black women with privileged class status are not exempt from this problem. The magazine of the Harvard School of Public Health described Serena Williams's case together with that of a fellow thirty-six-year-old elite Black woman, Shalon Irving, who was a PhD epidemiologist at the

CDC and yet died of complications a few weeks after giving birth.[22] Like many such accounts, the magazine piece describes a possible mechanism: the "weathering" that Black women experience as a result of living in a racist society, an increased allostatic load of stress that operates rather like premature aging.[23]

"Weathering" is a powerful concept that resonates with Black literary theorist Christina Sharpe's concept of "the weather": "the weather is the totality of our environments; the weather is the total climate; and that climate is antiblack."[24] The specific weather that individuals face is variable, and indeed the need to be adaptable in the face of changing weather conditions is itself a form of stress, but it is always inextricable from the context of a climate of anti-Black racism.

And yet the Harvard article's focal goal is not explanation but action: in the context of the U.S. medical system, it is not Black women's complicated health conditions that are the direct cause of the excess morbidity and mortality but the challenges in accessing care that could effectively treat those complications.[25] To put it into terms laid out in this book's introduction, if the differential rates of complications of pregnancy are the result of "the accumulated insults" of living in a racist society, their deadliness also comes from medical "inaction in the face of need."[26] For Shalon Irving, as was almost the case for Serena Williams, skepticism in the face of her description of her symptoms was a key locus of denial of care.

Anthropologist of racialization in childbirth Khiara Bridges discusses a report about inequity in treatment for childbirth complications as a contributor to maternal health disparities, which found that African American women are less likely to receive treatment for pregnancy-related hemorrhage even when the severity of bleeding was the same across racial groups. Bridges highlights the problematic explanation that the authors of the report provide for the unequal treatment: "In the case of post-partum haemorrhage, reluctance to report or under-reporting on the part of the patient or difference in history taking on the part of the physician could lead to differences in treatment for the same degree of hemorrhage."[27] Bridges suggests that the idea that Black women would be silent amid massive blood loss is implausible, reflective of "discourses of Black women's fantastical stoicism and strength," and that the "difference in history taking" should be named as physician racism.[28] In a way that is highly racially patterned, doctors are not listening to Black women.

When it comes to maternal health in the United States, even closing the racial disparities would not be enough. As neonatologist Richard David points out in the powerful documentary that explores the problem of Black women's and newborns' high levels of morbidity and mortality, "white Americans, if they were a separate country, [their infant mortality] would still rank 23rd in the world."[29] In this broken system, the women who are already most vulnerable are rendered more vulnerable still.

The high rate of C-sections may play a role in the riskiness of child-birth in the United States. Although the procedure can be life saving for both women and infants, it brings its own risks—for example, as in Serena Williams's case, the risk of internal bleeding. It is not clear why Williams's labor was induced in the first place—in her documentary series filmed for HBO Sports, all she says about it is that "the doctor said it was time, so I guess it was time"[30]—but induction often contributes to an escalation of medicalization. Market-driven health care is a key driver of the high C-section rate in the United States—from a hospital's perspective, surgical deliveries are both easier to manage in terms of scheduling and more lucrative in terms of payments.[31] Even Serena Wil-liams herself, speaking on the day that she went to the hospital to have her labor induced, seemed to be under the misapprehension that having a C-section "seems easier," though her doula corrected her—saying "not the recovery part!"[32] In her reflections on her pregnancy and childbirth experience in the documentary, Williams reflects, "I was so healthy, my pregnancy was so easy, like I didn't have any problems, but unfortunately, once I had the C-section, everything, from there, was pretty much a nightmare."[33] It is impossible to know what might have happened in her particular case had the birth not been induced and a C-section avoided, but broadly we can say that overuse of C-sections adversely impacts ma-ternal health, and Black women are even more likely than white women to undergo C-sections—a form of overtreatment that exacerbates risk in the face of systemic undertreatment. This reflects what Alondra Nelson has characterized as a central tension in the health inequality of African

Americans: poor Black communities have long been "both underserved by and overexposed to the medical system."[34]

HYPERVISIBILITY AND DEHUMANIZATION

In Serena Williams's articulation of her birth experience as a Black woman's experience, it is not Black women's bodies that are problematic; rather, it is the system that is, by failing to meet Black women's needs. This is an important intervention, because the field of obstetrics and gynecology is deeply implicated in the colonialist biopolitical paradigm that treats Black women's bodies as sites of extraction rather than of care. Marion Sims, hailed as the founder of gynecology, based his research on enslaved women, who were in turn configured as completely passive.[35] Exploiting myths about Black women's high tolerance for pain, Sims and his colleagues denied these women their full humanity even while treating them as ideal research subjects.[36] Although it may well be true that the enslaved women were eager for any care they could get for excruciating conditions such as fistula—even when that meant unanesthetized backyard surgeries—for Sims, the women were not treated as suffering patients in need. They were treated as damaged reproductive property, and because of their expendability, their bodies were for him promising terrain for the medical breakthroughs that would make him famous.

Sims's lack of deference to the pain of enslaved women is emblematic of the way that Black women's femininity itself was and is often thrown into question. It resonates with abolitionist and feminist Sojourner Truth's nineteenth-century provocation, in the face of white men's dismissal of equal rights for women on the grounds that women's delicacy required special care and her own experience of no such deference as a hardworking and abused enslaved woman, "ar'n't I a woman?"[37] If, ideologically, to be a woman is to receive accommodation and care, Black women's membership in the category of "woman" has never been universally sufficiently recognized. Even in today's biopolitical paradigm, denials of full citizenship and denials of femininity remain intertwined, and expendability and exploitability are linked.

The inherently political quality of the insistence on including Black women in the category of "woman" provides an opportunity to expand the scope from Williams's experience in childbirth and link that experience with the ways in which her broader life and career provide windows into the racialized denigration of Black women. Indeed, in some ways, Williams represents an extreme example of the denial of femininity to Black women. Invoking her muscularity and strength, internet abusers, among others, have gone so far as to question Serena Williams's status as female.[38] Throughout their careers, Serena and her sister Venus have faced accusations that their superior strength and physicality are somehow an unfair advantage: a 1998 article in the mass-market news magazine *Newsweek* stated that "American tennis legend Chris Evert says both sisters' athletic ability and raw aggression make it hard for 'the women who aren't Amazons' to compete with them."[39] Serena Williams, in particular, has been subjected to abuse online that has taunted her as "half man, half gorilla!," "built like an NFL linebacker," and more.[40] Like the Black South African runner Caster Semenya, whose appearance and performance prompted layers of sex testing, Serena Williams has been confronted with intertwined misogyny and racism that Black feminist health science studies scholar Moya Bailey has powerfully characterized as "misogynoir," a term that "describes the co-constitutive, anti-Black, and misogynistic racism directed at Black women, particularly in visual and digital culture."[41] Women athletes' femininity might always be in question to a certain degree, but for the Williams sisters, and especially for Serena, this derision has been inextricably bound to Blackness as well.[42]

Indeed, media representations have often simultaneously questioned the femininity of the Williams sisters while characterizing them—Serena Williams in particular—as too much of a woman, for displaying sexuality in ways inappropriate for the tennis court, an overwhelmingly elite white sport. The sexualized "grotesque" trope has led some Black feminist analysts and others to put Williams into the line of representation with the "Hottentot Venus" Saartjie Baartman, a South African woman who was displayed in London and Paris in the nineteenth century.[43] Those parodying Serena have emphasized large breasts and buttocks—notably her competitor (and friend) Danish player Caroline Wozniacki, who spurred controversy when she shoved towels down her shirt and skirt in a parody of Serena (a form of mocking in which white men have engaged as well).[44] The troubling of femininity that is going on in the obsession with large buttocks and breasts is different from the troubling of femininity that focuses on muscularity, because it is not evoking masculinity. However, this trope, too, is emblematic of distance from white feminine ideals.

Serena Williams has also been harshly criticized and occasionally penalized for expressing anger on the court.[45] She has been chided for "not keeping her head."[46] Because of the pervasiveness of stereotypes about "angry black women," this kind of approbation cannot be extricated from gender and race.[47] The fact that Williams rarely expresses anger off the court can be read as a strategy for navigating these stifling expectations.[48]

Representations of Serena Williams throughout her career can be understood as a paradoxical combination of hypervisibility and invisibility. She has long experienced surveillance of her body as a suspect category, an unbelievable Black body. Perhaps the most famous moment of this was the controversy around her 2002 Wimbledon "catsuit," which was both admired and derided as animalistic and sexy, displaying a combination of muscularity and curves that deviated from the lithe white feminine tennis norm.[49] Media representations of her body as emblematic of natural ability and yet deviant in terms of both gender and race have continued in coverage of tournaments for decades.[50] Her celebrity has not shielded her from ridicule.

It is worth noting that Serena Williams herself loved the catsuit and described it as "really innovative" and "sexy."[51] Williams can and does contest the ways that images of her are read. In this sense, Williams has been an unusually skilled navigator of the bind described by Black feminist sociologist Patricia Hill Collins:

> Surveillance operates via strategies of everyday racism whereby individual women feel that they are being "watched" in their desegregated work environments. Surveillance also functions via media representations that depict the success of selected high-achieving Black women. Surveillance seems designed to produce a particular effect—Black women remain

visible yet silenced; their bodies become written on by other texts, yet they remain powerless to speak for themselves.[52]

Even if it can be difficult to hear her voice amid the cacophony, Serena Williams certainly does speak for herself.

Postpregnancy, Williams wore another controversial catsuit to compete in the French Open, which covered not just her body but also her legs in a tight-fitting way designed to help with her blood-clotting issues. The appeal of the outfit was not exclusively medical—Serena made reference to the movie *Black Panther* as she told reporters, "I feel like a warrior in it, a warrior princess . . . from Wakanda, maybe," adding, "I've always wanted to be a superhero, and it's kind of my way of being a superhero."[53] Health and expression are not mutually exclusive—while noting that she herself had specific problems with blood clots that made wearing pants helpful to keep blood circulation going,[54] Williams dedicated the catsuit to "all the moms out there that had a tough pregnancy and have to come back and try to be fierce, in [the] middle of everything. That's what this represents."[55] The tournament officials responded by imposing a stricter dress code that would exclude such clothing going forward.

Yet even as she has repeatedly faced censure, Serena Williams's story of rising from humble beginnings through natural talent and hard work fits a particular narrative of the "American Dream," in which success can be achieved regardless of characteristics such as race, class, and gender.[56] This narrative of achieving the American Dream has helped to make Serena Williams's body ripe for commodification through advertising. Insofar as the success of the Williams sisters has been appropriated by the sport of tennis as symbolic of diversity and progress, it has also been used to let the Women's Tennis Association "off the hook" for its long-standing and ongoing lack of racial equality in the sport.[57]

NARRATIVE RETURN

For Serena Williams, tying her harrowing experience in childbirth to the experiences of other Black women marks something of a narrative return. Early in her career, when their father was a prominent spokesperson, the family often spoke about racism directly, most famously at Indian Wells in 2001, when the sisters were subjected to racial epithets and excessive booing from an angry crowd who suspected their father of match fixing, and went on to sit out that tournament for years.[58] As their careers developed, the Williams sisters shifted their focus in their public comments from talking about racism to trying to integrate themselves more—while still donating money to racial justice projects.[59]

By connecting her childbirth experience to those of other Black women, Serena Williams has come full circle. Whereas throughout her career, she has been in the white elite feminine space of tennis, in childbirth, she was in the white space of medicine. Tennis may be less segregated than it had been, but it has not escaped its elitist legacy. In the medical sphere, remaining exclusions are higher stakes. Many medical practitioners are not white, but they still participate in a structure that is fundamental to white supremacy. Williams's laboring body has been a resource for the spectacle of sport, but she has striven to maintain agency and voice. Her body in labor, she faced an analogous struggle.

In her voice-over on footage recorded by HBO Sports from the day that her labor was induced, Serena Williams reflected, "It shouldn't have been scary, going to the hospital to be induced. Or maybe it should have. But the more I think about it, fear has always been valuable in my life. Without fear, without doubt, without discomfort in what we are doing, what is there for any of us to overcome?"[60] She put that fear and overcoming into terms of taking on tennis opponents. But why should the experience of childbirth be similarly adversarial? Williams's husband, Alexis Ohanian, described his fear for her life in the HBO Sports documentary: "She was undoubtedly battling for her life, and I was terrified that she might die. But I was grateful that she had the wherewithal to speak because she knew her body better than any of us."[61]

Serena Williams advocating for herself in childbirth and speaking out about her experience thereafter highlights the political quality of Black women insisting on bodily well-being. As the important Black lesbian feminist poet, essayist, and memoirist Audre Lorde has famously argued, "caring for myself is not self-indulgence, it is self-preservation, and that is an act of political warfare."[62] In the contemporary era of the neoliberalization of "self-care," in which "care" denotes modest indulgences like spa treatments and bubble baths, it is easy to forget that when Lorde wrote her powerful statement, she was struggling with life-threatening liver cancer. Self-care can be life or death.

Within hours of Serena Williams's Facebook post describing her experience and highlighting the racial disparities in maternal mortality, stories from other women poured in to the comments. Serena Williams was moved, writing, "I'm in tears with all these stories I have almost read every single one of them—and plan on doing so! I'm glad we can speak out about this. Let's continue to let our voices be heard. That's the only way we can make change. <3 <3"

There are plenty of things that this kind of articulation leaves out. As important as it is to "let our voices be heard" as we share individual experiences, we can and should question whether that move itself is "the only way to make change." And yet there is something powerful in the mobilization of social media to share these personal stories, connect them to larger patterns of experience, and demand change. Serena Williams's sharing of her birth story in this way is an urgent contestation of the biopolitical paradigm that has rendered Black women's bodies expendable, and it offers an important locus for demanding full citizenship for Black women in both medical and public spheres.

In Serena Williams's decision to frame her experience along the lines of African American experience, we can see that intersections of race and biomedicine have an open-endedness to their mobilization. On one hand, biomedical ideas of race can be and in many spheres are used to maintain

Most Relevant ▾

Serena Williams ✓ I'm in tears with all these stories I have almost read every single one of them- and plan on doing so! I'm glad we can speak out about this. Let's continue to let our voices be heard. That's the only way to make change. 💙💙
2y   OO💙 1.1K

In this Facebook comment, Serena Williams describes herself as being in tears hearing other women's stories and urges women to continue to make their voices heard in order to make change. We see Williams's face from her profile image; that there are 87 comments; and that 1.1K people have reacted to the post with "like," "love," and "wow." Facebook comment by Serena Williams. Screen grab by Katherine Behar.

historically entrenched ideas about race—for example, arguing that op-pressed racialized groups are somehow inherently and essentially inferior. Yet this is a site in which we can see race in medicine being mobilized in the other direction: to stake a claim to the right to full citizenship and health and to resist race-based injustice. As exceptional as Serena Wil-liams is, her birth story and the dissemination and mobilization of that story on social media and beyond have much to offer for advocacy for reproductive justice.

Conclusion

As I write this in the long lockdown summer of 2020 in London, little seems more routine than scrolling through my social media feed. For months, my feed seemed to be all COVID-19, all the time—at first a jumble of frantically shared, haphazardly assessed epidemiological reports, interspersed with personal stories of friends' struggles in lockdown and fears of getting sick or transmitting illness, and later increasingly expressions of mounting frustration at political leaders for their poor management of the crisis and talk of the U.S. elections ahead. Yet occasionally, events of a different tenor joined the feed: outrageous murders of Black people—the vigilante killing of jogger Ahmaud Arbery in Georgia in February, the video of which was released in May; the police killing of Breonna Taylor in her own Kentucky home as she slept in March; and especially the police murder of George Floyd in May, caught on video, a white police officer constraining him with a knee on his neck, other officers standing by, as Floyd pleaded, "I can't breathe."

The sharing of outrage over these specific events marked a return to and intensification of a pervasive element of social media before the novel coronavirus crisis: accounts of harassment and violence against racialized minorities, especially Black people. And the events keep coming—unexplained murders of Black trans women, white women calling the police on Black people for minor or nonexistent infractions, and killings of unarmed Black people by police and vigilantes. As Black Lives Matter activists have highlighted, these are examples of phenomena that are absolutely routine. These events should provoke our outrage precisely because they are all too ordinary.

These events deserve sustained attention. Unpacking their specificities can reveal a great deal about the particular interlocking structures that shape our unequal world. A fundamental contention of this book has been that our analysis should *begin* with the outrage at these events and their ubiquity; it should not *end* there. We need to go beyond holding such events up as fundamentally interchangeable examples of a world gone wrong.

There is value in sitting a little longer than a news cycle with the events that spur these moments of outrage. Stories of suffering can be so much cacophony in our social media feeds and in our collective consciousness. Amid the scrolling, poignant accounts of racism and other forms of oppression can and should spur outrage, and also insight. To be analytically meaningful, individual experiences cannot and should not be isolated from the social structure in which they emerge. A story isolated from its context is at best an anecdote. By itself, no small experience or event that I describe is convincing proof of the structure at work. An individual story can *illustrate* structural inequality, but broader social inquiry is necessary to *demonstrate* structural inequality. Moreover, what might seem like disparate events can and should be usefully read together. Deep engagement with past events can equip us analytically to confront current and future crises.

CONNECTING 2020 WITH THE EVENTS
AND THEMES OF THIS BOOK

Each event described in this book has distinctive resonances with this time of COVID-19 and intensified anger over police violence. This book was largely written before the crisis of the novel coronavirus that causes COVID-19 and the contemporaneous global resurgence of the Black Lives Matter movement. Yet the book's account can be helpful for beginning to grapple with both the racially disparate impact of the disease and the highly visible instances of police and vigilante violence that have spurred anger and activism. Here, I consider resonances between the cases that I have analyzed from the first two decades of the twenty-first century and the events of 2020 to offer an opportunity to reflect on events past, present, and future.

Sickening began with a chapter considering another moment of twinned crises in which Americans were initially figured as newly vulnerable and "all in this together" in the face of a global threat: the deaths of Black postal workers in the 2001 anthrax attacks very soon after the terrorist attacks of September 11. In a largely forgotten audio precursor to the viral videos that have been iconic of the Black Lives Matter era, one postal worker's 911 call recorded shortly before he died provided an account of the structural and personally mediated racism that would lead to his death: a refusal by his governmental employers to acknowledge, address, or communicate about the dangers of (what we would now call) the "essential work" of sorting and delivering the mail, followed by inaction in the face of individual need by his health care provider, who failed to take his illness seriously. The sense that twenty-first-century terrorism was novel in terms of the scale with which it endangered Americans "at home" obscured the fact that it rendered particularly vulnerable those within the U.S. body politic who were never safe—not before 9/11, not after.

The focus of the second chapter was another crisis of American identity and unity: the racially disparate impact of Hurricane Katrina, in which the fissures in the body politic have been more widely recognized than they were in the wake of 9/11. The largely poor and Black population of New Orleans had been made acutely vulnerable by the governmental expectation that people would pursue safety on their own. The orders to evacuate the city in advance of the storm were impossible to follow for many who did not have access to either private cars or any other form of transportation, in a way that is evocative of the impossibility of following the COVID-era orders to "shelter in place" for those who must leave home to support their household's basic needs. Criminalization of those who were either going about their lives or seeking help—gathering food from shuttered supermarkets, or those seeking shelter in the Superdome—resonates with police and vigilante violence that is so pervasive today. At the same time, media preoccupation with "looters" obscures structural violence. As in the current crisis, long-standing structurally induced heightened burdens of chronic diseases, such as cardiovascular disease and diabetes, made African Americans more vulnerable still to acute illness. Now, as then, the fragmented and inadequate U.S. health care system compounds the harms of baseline exclusions.

Mass incarceration was the focus of the third chapter, on the suspended sentences of the Scott sisters. Mass incarceration has been foregrounded in both of the twinned crises of the current moment as well: excessive imprisonment enacted through a structurally racist criminal justice system goes hand in hand with harms to the bodies of prisoners themselves. The racially disparate harm to health that mass incarceration instantiates is not new to this extraordinary time, and yet attention to the extraordinary can meaningfully illuminate the routine violence of prisons as institutions that contribute to the constitution of contemporary racialization and the denial of full citizenship. Prisons and jails have been sites of some of the largest coronavirus outbreaks, rendering people who are awaiting trial or who have been convicted of crimes, whether serious or trivial, particularly vulnerable to exposure. In a way that is similar to "essential workers" but even more heightened, prisoners are treated as disposable. Even when the illnesses and deaths are technically due to a disease, the source of the suffering should be located as the system. Calls for prison abolition have become increasingly urgent.

The fourth chapter highlights the stratification of environmental and infrastructural risk in the preferential treatment of General Motors' machines over the population of Flint in that city's infamous water crisis. This, too, is relevant in the current moment. For example, an extraordinary number of households in nearby Detroit have lacked access to running water because their services had been shut off for being behind on onerous water bill payments—and this human rights violation has extra impact in a pandemic, by making it impossible for people to follow hygiene guidance.[1] More broadly, the austerity-induced scarcity of infrastructural capacity in particular places is too often taken for granted. Decades of disinvestment in public health infrastructure have created a terrain in which bodies are differentially vulnerable to heightened precarity. The Flint water crisis took place in the context of the imposition of emergency financial management, prioritizing bond holders over residents, which was bad for health generally and particularly bad for African Americans. As in postcolonial contexts in which structural adjustment policies have been imposed, prioritization of the financial sector over the survivability of people exemplifies biopolitical inequalities.

A primary focus of the fifth chapter, on the McKinney pool party incident, is police brutality as a mechanism by which segregation is enforced. The violent control of access to leisure has been a foregrounded element of this moment, in which we have been urged to "stay home" in unequal homes and socially distanced outdoor space has not been available to all. Another focus was the role of professional media in the civil rights movement and amateur social media today. The McKinney pool party case was a relatively early example of the kinds of viral videos that have catalyzed Black Lives Matter and have gained in importance since then. In a way that is both continuous and discontinuous with the way that images were created and distributed in the twentieth-century civil rights movement, amateur videographers and artists have generated and distributed images of police violence in their demands for justice.

The sixth chapter, on Serena Williams's birth story, returns to the fundamental issue of denial of care that was highlighted in the first chapter. Black communities and individuals are hypersurveilled but inadequately cared for. The concept of "weathering," invoked to understand the premature aging caused by living in a racist society that has impact on maternal health and birth outcomes, might also be evocative for understanding heightened Black vulnerability to COVID at younger ages. Self-advocacy is important but is also not enough, as health care providers all too often do not listen to or trust Black patients. In the mobilization of Williams's story for reproductive justice advocacy, as in the mobilization of stories of COVID-19 and of police violence for Black Lives Matter, we can also see community strength and resilience in the contestation of oppression.

More broadly, each chapter highlights the vitality of biopolitical questions of racism and health disparities that are so urgent in the current moment—within the body politic, whose lives are fostered, and whose are not? Importantly, the ethical scope of this question must not be limited to the intensive care unit. Rationing of health care resources is not new to COVID times. If many people have become newly afraid of rationing, that is because they had scant prior awareness that there were already segments of the population who had routinely been left out of the allocation of care. I hope that this book also points to the need to move beyond "lifeboat ethics" in the coronavirus context and more generally.[2]

In coronavirus times, there has been more interest in discussing the al-location of mechanical ventilators than in questioning the conditions that made some bodies more vulnerable than others in the first place. We can and should decry the unequal provision of medical care, in crisis times and in ordinary times, and we should also illuminate how wide-ranging elements of the social world beyond health care settings contribute to the stratification of health and well-being.

THE SICKENING ASSIGNMENT: A TEMPLATE FOR ANALYSIS

There are many compelling cases of racism and health disparities beyond what I have been able to analyze here, and there will undoubtedly be more in the future. How might readers carry out a similar form of analysis in the face of social injustices that occur in different times and places? Here, I outline an activity along the lines of assignments that I have developed for my own undergraduate classrooms.[3] This four-step template can be adapted for use in wide-ranging classroom contexts or engaged by readers to guide them in writing their own analyses.

1. Map out the Terrain: Look across Scales
    Find a Micro Scale: Sometimes the intimate scale is already pres-ent in a case as it is disseminated in the media—there is an event that happened to a specific, named person, in a particular encounter at a particular moment in time. Thus, the micro scale might be a very specific first-person account, as here with the postal worker's 911 call. Other times, however, the analyst will have to be creative to pick out and highlight a small element within a larger event—for example, the ability of General Motors to protect its engine plant during the Flint water crisis. In this scale, you might find a combination of institution-alized racism, personally mediated racism, and internalized racism.[4]
    Find a Meso Scale: Attend to the surroundings of the event. What is the near context in which this event occurs, chronologically and socially? In what kind of space—neighborhood/city/region—does the event occur, and how does that matter? Who else is around, whether as participant or bystander? The meso scale might be a city or a suburb, an

organization or a social sphere, each associated with particular health care systems and systems of social control. This scale will often reveal institutionalized racism.

Find a Macro Scale: Attend to the broader social and historical context of the event. How does it emerge out of trends in history and society in the United States (or other national context)? How does it participate in the political economy of the contemporary health care system and the entrenched biopolitical priorities that render some lives differentially disposable? How does it reflect major drivers of racial inequality, such as the structures of segregation, access to care, and exposure to harms? This scale is vital for attending to institutionalized racism.

2. Inform Your Account: Read

Read Media Closely: Newspapers, magazines, and social media posts do more than present an account of an event; they shape stories and provide broader narratives. Attend not only to what they are saying but also to how they are saying it. What is assumed about the readers of the story, including their background assumptions, default sympathies, and emotional responses? Who is presented as the protagonist of the story, who is in the background, and who is rendered invisible? Whose interests are treated as urgent sites of concern? Whose conditions of privilege or deprivation are taken for granted and treated as the normal state of affairs? How are the people involved articulated as full members of the "American public" (or not)?

Read Materials from Activist Organizations: This overlaps with reading media broadly, since both mainstream and activist accounts are often featured in social media, blogs, and online magazines. But it is important to be intentional about finding sources that are explicitly engaged in advocating for justice. How are those who are mobilizing around the case framing what has happened, and to what ends?

Read Relevant Scholarship: Scholarly writing is invaluable for grappling in a rigorous way with history and broader social context. Scholarly writing is easy to identify: broadly, it is written by people who have academic affiliations—that is, their bylines will say their title (such as PhD student or professor) and institution (such as a university or research organization) rather than merely "writer"—and it cites its sources, including referring to what other scholars have said. Note: make sure that your reading includes work by Black scholars (this will come up again below).

3. Enrich Your Analytical Frame: Add Layers of Analysis

Pay Attention to History: Look beyond the flash of the news cycle and search for ways in which the contemporary event emerges out of a history.[5]

Pay Attention to Infrastructure: How is the built environment contributing to the situation in which the event transpires? What about systems of distribution of goods and services?

Pay Attention to Technology: Some of the technologies that I have discussed are obviously medical—pharmaceuticals, especially. Yet many technologies that matter are not medical, ranging from pipes to swimming pools to cell phone cameras.

Pay Attention to Economic Context: Who is working, and how are they paid? Who is paying for things, how are they doing so, and who benefits? How does capitalism matter?

Pay Attention to Citizenship Claims: Who is in a position to make demands of the state and of other powerful institutions, including but not limited to medical institutions? How do they make those demands, and in the face of what resistance?

Pay Attention to Intersections: Race is not the only category of identity at stake in any particular experience or event. Pay attention to how race intersects with class, gender, age, disability, sexuality, and other systems of power.

Pay Attention to Voice: Whose stories are being represented in the dominant account? How might you seek out additional, less prominent perspectives?

Pay Attention to Knowledge: Start local: how have you come to know about the event? But also pay attention to the ways that knowledge matters in the event: whose knowledge is valued, whose is discounted, who is treated as an expert, who is believed at all, and how does it matter?

Pay Attention to Power: Who has it, and how is it used? Who doesn't have it, and how does it matter?

4. Write Your Account

Remember the Humanity: Sometimes the people whose stories are invoked become lost behind a slogan. Be sure to recount the stories with compassion. The system is brutal, but your treatment of the subjects should not be.

Remember Social Justice: Sometimes the story of the individual is so compelling that it makes it hard to see the terrain. Attending to individual human experiences of suffering is not an alternative to attending to structural oppression but a necessary complement to it. Moreover, analysis of racism should not simply be an intellectual exercise but should always be oriented toward justice.[6]

Cite Black Women: "Cite Black Women" is a hashtag and a website (http://www.citeblackwomen.org/), and it is also a call to practice.[7] No matter what your own identity is, it is absolutely vital to read Black women's media production and scholarship. If the event at the center of your analysis is about the experiences of another racialized group, such as Indigenous people or non-Black immigrants, also seek out scholarly and activist accounts by people who are members of that group. This does not mean that you must *exclusively* cite Black women and other scholars of color.[8] But any account—especially but not only about topics like racism and health—will be hopelessly empty without engaging with what Black women have already written. Moreover, give credit to those Black women writers in your own account.

Although these steps are numbered 1–4, they are necessarily iterative. Reading will help to articulate scales for analysis, curiosity about additional layers of analysis will spur additional research, and the writing process is itself inextricable from the analysis. Working through the components once might get an analysis started, but creating a compelling account will require working through the stories and analytical frames multiple times over.

I have elaborated this analytical template with attention to racism and health in the contemporary United States in mind, but readers may also find it useful for analysis of other topics, times, and places. I have endeavored to make the components concrete enough to be feasibly realized as described, even as I offer them with the understanding and expectation that teachers and readers will make modifications for their own contexts, circumstances, and focal concerns.

The chapters of this book have provided examples of this template in action. My approach has involved attending to wide-ranging contexts and analyzing cases across scales. This book has looked at harms to health that have occurred across different domains: workplaces, communities, prisons, environments, leisure spaces, health care settings. Those harms have been diverse: infectious disease, chronic disease, kidney failure, lead poisoning, bodily constraint, maternal mortality. Their impacts have been borne on different scales as well: by individuals, their workplaces, communities, families, cities. I hope that my accounts of each event, and how the range of events work together, provide analytical insight into each of the particular instances and into the broader patterns of personally mediated and especially institutionalized racism. Different cases will spur distinctive lines of inquiry, and I hope that the diversity of my own examples is generative.

TAKE (ADDITIONAL) ACTION

Analysis is important—it helps us to make sense of human experience and to understand the social world in which we live. Other forms of action matter too. It is beyond the scope of this book to describe precisely what actions readers should take to address the injustices analyzed here, but I hope that this book spurs curiosity to explore opportunities to get involved with such efforts. Moreover, I hope that the diversity of stories has helped to highlight the wide-ranging domains in which readers might take additional action.

The chapters have included many examples of people taking action against racism in health in wide-ranging ways. Some of the actions have taken place on an intimate, interpersonal scale of advocating and caring for family members and patients. Others have taken place in broader social spheres, raising awareness about injustice and demanding change. This has sometimes been undertaken by people acting individually and then amplifying their stories through social media: a teen with a cell phone camera recording police violence at a pool party, a celebrity recounting the barriers she faced accessing urgently needed medical care for complications of childbirth. Important work has also been done by groups of people in many kinds of organizations—the Association of Black Cardiologists advocating for victims of Hurricane Katrina; the Malcolm X Grassroots Movement and Black church groups mobilizing against the unjust incarceration of the Scott sisters; SisterSong Women of Color Reproductive Justice Collective working to empower Black women "to maintain personal bodily autonomy, have children, not have children, and parent the children we have in safe and sustainable communities."[9]

If you aren't already involved, it can be hard to know where to begin, but if you start looking, you can find a point of entry. Get involved where you find yourself. If you are a student or an educator, look for groups working on these issues at your school, college, or university. Whether you are academically affiliated or not, look for groups in your neighborhood, city, and region as well. Reading and perhaps further reflection on your own experiences have, hopefully, equipped you with some baseline understanding, but as you get involved wherever you are, start by listening and learning from what is already going on, rather than just charging in. You likely will have something to contribute, but you won't be able to know what that might be until you've listened to the ongoing conversations and seen the initiatives already under way.

There are many places to find these already existing endeavors. You might start with direct action groups, such as a Black Lives Matter chapter if you happen to have one in your city, or another group working for racial justice.[10] Another good place to start is with local governance—start following local news, keeping an eye out for relevant issues on the docket of the city council or similar body, and show up when people are speaking at a hearing. Those speakers can alert you to organizations and initiatives with which you might connect. Other institutions, such as libraries and especially independent Black and feminist bookstores, also often provide entrees—look for events and meetings there, and attend them. Artistic and cultural events with political content, too, can be excellent starting points.

The opportunities for involvement will be different in each locality, but my experience in Atlanta might be illustrative. I started to find my political community there when meeting organizers at a workshop held at the MondoHomo queer music and arts festival. That led to participating in mobilization against a particular proposed law that would have intensified criminalization of street-level sex workers, which led to contributing to the development of the transformative organization Solutions Not Punishment.[11] I also found and contributed to intersectional feminist community by serving on the board of the feminist bookstore Charis Books & More.[12] Along the way, I worked with other faculty in support of antiracist and other social justice advocacy on my university campus. As this list illustrates, my preference is for the local—if you are more drawn to national politics, you can start by getting involved in national campaigns for candidates you believe in; if you are more drawn to global social movements, you can start by connecting with those. Many people find like-minded community with which to organize through social media—find out who to follow, and start to get involved.

There is also scope for action against racism in health within health care. Those who currently work in health fields—or are in the process of training to work in health fields—can challenge themselves to work against the medical system's deeply ingrained biases against trusting Black patients in need. They can also work for transformation from within, such as physicians practicing "structural competency"[13] or doulas supporting Black women in childbirth.[14] Those working in medical fields also have a special role in advocacy against the structural inequalities in health care delivery—they can advocate for authentically universal access to care, both in theory and in practice—and for the diminishment of structural inequalities more broadly.[15] Medical practitioners, including those in training, can also put their esteemed standing to use by taking part in direct action, through organizations such as White Coats for Black Lives.[16]

As each of the chapters of this book and the COVID-19 crisis have demonstrated, medical systems are one urgent site of change. Martin Luther King Jr.'s famous 1966 clarion call against segregation in health care remains resonant today: "of all the forms of inequality, injustice in health is the most shocking and inhuman."[17] King was talking about the harms of segregated hospitals, but throughout his life of advocacy, he highlighted the need for much broader transformation. All citizens, and indeed all residents, can also work for change in diverse domains.

The racially disparate impact of the coronavirus and the intensified mobilization against police and vigilante violence of 2020 have underscored the urgent need for transformation in and beyond health care. Health care institutions are urgent targets for action, but they are not the only ones. Health is more than a medical matter.[18] Legal structures that privilege profit over people can be changed. Housing policies and structures that reinforce segregation can be redesigned. Police and prison systems can be made more accountable to public concern—or abolished. Another world is possible.

Notes

INTRODUCTION

1. Ruha Benjamin, *Race after Technology* (Cambridge: Polity Press, 2019), 13.
2. Benjamin, 15.
3. World Health Organization, http://apps.who.int/gb/bd/PDF/bd48/basic-documents-48th-edition-en.pdf#page=7.
4. Adam M. Geary, *Anti-Black Racism and the AIDS Epidemic* (New York: Palgrave Macmillan, 2014). The invisibility of Black women with AIDS that Evelynn M. Hammonds highlighted much earlier in the epidemic continues. Hammonds, "Missing Persons: Black Women and AIDS," *Radical America* 24, no. 2 (1990): 7–24.
5. The resonances may be particularly strong for those reading from other settler-colonial contexts in which anti-Black racism is foundational to the social milieu, such as Brazil and South Africa. See work by scholars working in and on those regions, including Melissa S. Creary, "Biocultural Citizenship and Embodying Exceptionalism: Biopolitics for Sickle Cell Disease in Brazil," *Social Science and Medicine* 199 (2018): 123–31; Zimitri Erasmus, *Race Otherwise: Forging a New Humanism for South Africa* (Johannesburg: Wits University Press, 2017).
6. See, e.g., the rich two-volume work of W. Michael Byrd and Linda A. Clayton, *An American Health Dilemma: A Medical History of African Americans and the Problem of Race, Beginnings to 1900* (New York: Routledge, 2000) and *An American Health Dilemma: Vol. II. Race, Medicine, and Health Care in the United States 1900–2000* (New York: Routledge, 2002). Even books with "twenty-first century" in the title, such as Dorothy Roberts's important *Fatal Invention: How Science, Politics, and Big Business Re-create Race in the Twenty-First Century* (New York: New Press, 2012), narrate the story chronologically from that same earlier foundation.
7. The scholarship of the Tuskegee Syphilis Study is robust, and rich points of entry might be either the foundational volume by James H.

Jones, *Bad Blood: The Tuskegee Syphilis Experiment* (New York: Free Press, 1981), or the more recent edited collection Susan M. Reverby, ed., *Tuskegee's Truths: Rethinking the Tuskegee Syphilis Study* (Chapel Hill: University of North Carolina Press, 2012). The Henrietta Lacks case came to prominence with the publication of Rebecca Skloot's *The Immortal Life of Henrietta Lacks* (New York: Crown, 2010), and it had long been a subject of interest to historians interested in the ways that biotechnologies have intersected with notions of race and racial exploitation. See Hannah Landecker, "Immortality, In Vitro: A History of the HeLa Cell Line," in *Biotechnology and Culture: Bodies, Anxieties, Ethics,* ed. Paul Brodwin, 53–72 (Bloomington: Indiana University Press, 2000).

8. The term *slow violence* comes from Rob Nixon, *Slow Violence and the Environmentalism of the Poor* (Cambridge, Mass.: Harvard University Press, 2011).

9. See, e.g., Jonathan Kahn, *Race in a Bottle: The Story of BiDil and Racialized Medicine in a Post-genomic Age* (New York: Columbia University Press, 2012); Roberts, *Fatal Invention,* 2. Many books that take a specifically more biological (as opposed to medical) frame also more justifiably use this same event as a hook, including Jenny Reardon, *The Postgenomic Condition: Ethics, Knowledge, and Justice after the Genome* (Chicago: University of Chicago Press, 2017), 2; Ian Whitmarsh and David S. Jones, *What's the Use of Race? Modern Governance and the Biology of Difference* (Cambridge, Mass.: MIT Press, 2010), 2.

10. There have been many debunkings of genetics as a driver of health disparities—see, e.g., Pamela Sankar, Mildred K. Cho, Celeste M. Condit, Linda M. Hunt, Barbara Koenig, Patricia Marshall, Sandra Soo-Jin Lee, and Paul Spicer, "Genetic Research and Health Disparities," *Journal of the American Medical Association* 291, no. 24 (2004): 2985–89. More recent commentary has reiterated the frame and the debunking: Kathleen McGlone West, Erika Blacksher, and Wylie Burke, "Genomics, Health Disparities, and Missed Opportunities for the Nation's Research Agenda," *Journal of the American Medical Association* 317, no. 18 (2017): 1831–32. See also physical anthropologist Clarence C. Gravlee's important work on how racism *produces* biological difference, in ways that are not genetically deterministic, in Gravlee, "How Race Becomes Biology: Embodiment of Social Inequality," *American Journal of Physical Anthropology* 139, no. 1 (2009): 47–57.

11. Cf. Wendy Hui Kyong Chun, "Race and/as Technology, or How to Do

Things to Race," in *Race after the Internet,* ed. Lisa Nakamura and Peter Chow-White, 44–66 (New York: Routledge, 2013).

12. The concept of "durability" has been developed further in my prior work. See Anne Pollock, *Medicating Race: Heart Disease and Durable Preoccupations with Difference* (Durham, N.C.: Duke University Press, 2012), esp. 8–12.

13. Camara Phyllis Jones, Benedict I. Truman, Laurie D. Elam-Evans, Camille A. Jones, Clara Y. Jones, Ruth Jiles, Susan F. Rumisha, and Geraldine S. Perry, "Using 'Socially Assigned Race' to Probe White Advantages in Health Status," *Ethnicity and Disease* 18 (2008): 496–504.

14. Barbara J. Fields, "AHR Forum of Rogues and Geldings," *American Historical Review* 108, no. 5 (2003): 1397–1405.

15. See, e.g., Kimberlé Crenshaw, "Mapping the Margins: Intersectionality, Identity Politics, and Violence against Women of Color," *Stanford Law Review* 43, no. 6 (1991): 1241–99. Terminology is explicitly discussed on p. 1244 in note 6: "I use 'Black' and 'African American' interchangeably throughout this article. I capitalize 'Black' because 'Blacks,' like Asians, Latinos, and other 'minorities,' constitute a specific cultural group and, as such, require denotation as a proper noun. . . . By the same token, I do not capitalize 'white,' which is not a proper noun, since whites do not constitute a specific cultural group. For the same reason I do not capitalize 'women of color.'" Others have raised legitimate problems with capitalizing *Black,* especially around the danger of naturalizing and reifying the category—with such a fraught concept, all terminology is problematic, and the predominant convention in antiracist scholarship is my main guide.

16. Of course, it is perfectly possible to combine interest in the social processes with interest in the individual psychologies of those navigating the racist society—canonically, see Frantz Fanon, *Black Skin, White Masks* (London: Paladin, 1970), esp. his reflections in chapter 5, "The Fact of Blackness" (109–16), on an encounter with a French child who exclaims, "Look, a Negro!"

17. Evelynn M. Hammonds, "New Technologies of Race," in *Processed Lives: Gender and Technology in Everyday Life,* ed. Jennifer Terry and Melodie Calvert, 107–22 (New York: Routledge, 1997).

18. Camara Phyllis Jones, "Levels of Racism: A Theoretic Framework and a Gardener's Tale," *American Journal of Public Health* 90, no. 8 (2000): 1212–13.

19. Zinzi D. Bailey, Nancy Krieger, Madina Agénor, Jasmine Graves, Natalia

Linos, and Mary T. Bassett, "Structural Racism and Health Inequities in the USA: Evidence and Interventions," *The Lancet* 389, no. 10077 (2017): 1453–63.

20. See David S. Jones, *Rationalizing Epidemics: Meanings and Uses of American Indian Mortality since 1600* (Cambridge, Mass.: Harvard University Press, 2004).

21. For a reader that is particularly rich in its inclusion of attention to Latino as well as Black health disparities, see Laurie B. Green, John Mckiernan-Gonzalez, and Martin Summers, eds., *Precarious Prescriptions: Contested Histories of Race and Health in North America* (Minneapolis: University of Minnesota Press, 2014).

22. Jonathan M. Metzl, *Dying of Whiteness: How the Politics of Racial Resentment Is Killing America's Heartland* (New York: Basic Books, 2019).

23. For further discussion, see Pollock, *Medicating Race,* esp. 96–97.

24. Intersectionality is a foundational concept in Black feminist theory, and although it is particularly useful for analyzing intragroup differences (the specificity of Black women's experiences, for example, which are not the same as Black men's experiences), it also helps to attend to the inextricability of multiple facets of identity. Crenshaw, "Mapping the Margins."

25. Nancy Krieger, "Embodying Inequality: A Review of Concepts, Measures, and Methods for Studying Health Consequences of Discrimination," *International Journal of Health Services* 29, no. 2 (1999): 295–352. The term *accumulated insults* is laid out in the abstract on p. 295 and on p. 296. For elaboration of how inequality becomes embodied as "the social *produces* the biological in a system of constant feedback between body and social experience," see Anne Fausto-Sterling, "The Bare Bones of Race," *Social Studies of Science* 38, no. 5 (2008): 657–94.

26. Michel Foucault, *The History of Sexuality Volume 1: An Introduction,* trans. Robert Hurley (1978; repr., New York: Vintage, 1990), 138.

27. Janet Shim, "Bio-power and Racial, Class, and Gender Formation in Biomedical Knowledge Production," *Research in the Sociology of Health Care* 17 (2000): 174.

28. See, e.g., Nikolas Rose, *The Politics of Life Itself: Biomedicine, Power, and Subjectivity in the Twenty-First Century* (Princeton, N.J.: Princeton University Press, 2007), esp. chapter 6, "Race in the Age of Genomic Medicine" (155–86).

29. Anthony Ryan Hatch, *Blood Sugar: Racial Pharmacology and Food Justice in Black America* (Minneapolis: University of Minnesota Press, 2016), 17.

30. Shiloh Krupar and Nadine Ehlers, "Biofutures: Race and the Governance of Health," *Environment and Planning D: Society and Space* 35, no. 2 (2017): 222–40; Jonathan Xavier Inda, *Racial Prescriptions: Pharmaceuticals, Difference, and the Politics of Life* (New York: Routledge, 2016).

31. Nadine Ehlers and Shiloh Krupar, *Deadly Biocultures: The Ethics of Life-making* (Minneapolis: University of Minnesota Press, 2019). The overview of Foucauldian biopower appears on pp. 2–5 and leads to the elaboration of "deadly life-making" on pp. 5–7.

32. Melissa Harris-Perry, *Sister Citizen: Shame, Stereotypes, and Black Women in America* (New Haven, Conn.: Yale University Press, 2011), 4.

33. Melissa Harris-Perry gave a virtuosic keynote address at a conference on "Politics of Health in the U.S. South" (Vanderbilt University, March 17, 2016), in which she evocatively framed Black Lives Matter in terms of that theme. She gave the provocation that has stayed with me since: that we understand politics as matter, health as lives, and the U.S. South as Black.

34. Classic examples include Steven Shapin and Simon Schaffer, *Leviathan and the Air-Pump: Hobbes, Boyle, and the Experimental Life* (Princeton, N.J.: Princeton University Press, 1985); Bruno Latour, *Science in Action: How to Follow Scientists and Engineers through Society* (Cambridge, Mass.: Harvard University Press, 1988).

35. For discussion, see John Law, "STS as Method," in *The Handbook of Science and Technology Studies,* ed. Ulrike Felt, Rayvon Fouché, Clark Miller, and Laurel Smith-Doerr, 31–58 (Cambridge, Mass.: MIT Press, 2016).

36. Donna Haraway has long read media together with scientific texts; see, e.g., Haraway, *Simians, Cyborgs, and Women: The Reinvention of Nature* (New York: Routledge, 1991).

37. Indeed, there is room to go further and include deeper engagement with fiction. See Ruha Benjamin, "Racial Fictions, Biological Facts: Expanding the Sociological Imagination through Speculative Methods," *Catalyst: Feminism, Theory, Technoscience* 2, no. 2 (2016).

38. Mary G. McDonald and Susan Birrell, "Reading Sport Critically: A Methodology for Interrogating Power," *Sociology of Sport Journal* 16, no. 4 (1999): 283–300.

39. This is following in the footsteps of, e.g., Moya Bailey, "Misogynoir in Medical Media: On Caster Semenya and R. Kelly," *Catalyst: Feminism, Theory, Technoscience* 2, no. 2 (2016).

40. Moya Bailey and Whitney Peoples, "Articulating Black Feminist Health Science Studies," *Catalyst: Feminism, Theory, Technoscience* 3, no. 2 (2017).

41. Nassim Parvin, "Doing Justice to Stories: On Ethics and Politics of Digital Storytelling," *Engaging Science, Technology, and Society* 4 (2018): 515–34.
42. See, e.g., the important work of medical sociologists who use novel interviews to show how structural inequality shapes experiences of such wide-ranging phenomena as cardiovascular disease and autism. On cardiovascular disease, see Janet K. Shim, *Heart-sick: The Politics of Risk, Inequality, and Heart Disease* (New York: NYU Press, 2014). On autism, see Jennifer Singh, who explores the little-studied topic of barriers to autism services for single Black mothers and grandmothers. Alice Hong and Jennifer Singh, "Contextualizing the Social and Structural Constraints of Accessing Autism Services among Single Black Female Caregivers," *International Journal of Child Health and Human Development* 12, no. 4 (2020): 365–78. Many additional examples are referenced throughout this book.

1. TERRORISM

1. All of the 911 quotes interspersed in the text are from the transcript of the call Morris made at 4:39 A.M., October 21, 2001. The full text was released by the Associated Press, November 8, 2001. Others have also drawn on this powerful transcript for political commentary, notably including imprisoned activist Mumia Abu-Jamal, "Powerless at the Post Office," *Michigan Citizen,* December 29, 2001, V.XXIV, no. 5 A7.
2. There is one notable account of the impact of racism on health that does include a several-page discussion of this case, in the context of the failure of the government to provide equal body protection to African Americans, in a chapter on "Separate and Unequal Treatment: Response to Health Emergencies, Human Experiments, and Bioterrorism Threats," under the evocative subheading "Will Government Response to Bioterrorism Be Fair?," in Robert D. Bullard and Beverly Wright, *The Wrong Complexion for Protection: How the Government Response to Disaster Endangers African American Communities,* 197–201 (New York: NYU Press, 2012).
3. The Tuskegee Syphilis Study has been the subject of a considerable body of scholarship; good entry points might be either the foundational volume by Jones, *Bad Blood,* or the more recent edited collection by Reverby, *Tuskegee's Truths.*
4. References to Tuskegee were a recurring theme in focus groups of

Brentwood postal workers reflecting on communication during the anthrax crisis. Janice C. Blanchard, Yolanda Haywood, Bradley D. Stein, Terri L. Tanielian, Michael Stoto, and Nicole Lurie, "In Their Own Words: Lessons Learned from Those Exposed to Anthrax," *American Journal of Public Health* 95, no. 3 (2005): 489–95.

5. Ruha Benjamin, "Organized Ambivalence: When Sickle Cell Disease and Stem Cell Research Converge," *Ethnicity and Health* 16, no. 4–5 (2011): 447.

6. I have been unable to find sufficient information about the other survivors to include them in this chapter. One, whose daughter gave an interview without releasing his name, went to the ER on October 25 while feeling relatively mild symptoms for two days (nausea and tiring easily) because two of his coworkers had already died and his job includes sorting government mail. He described his job in detail to the physician there, and he pressed for and received one tablet of Cipro pending his swab results. He returned twenty-four hours later as instructed and was promptly aggressively treated. He was released after sixteen days and wants to remain unnamed. Jennifer Lenhart, "Anthrax Patient Is 'Just So Tired' Va. Mail Worker Making Progress," *Washington Post,* November 9, 2001.

7. Tom Daschle, "The Unsolved Case of Anthrax," *Washington Post,* October 15, 2006.

8. Courtland Miloy, "Anthrax Mystery and Misery Linger for Postal Workers," *Washington Post,* October 25, 2006.

9. Jill Nelson, "The Façade of National Unity," MSNBC Opinions, http://stacks.msnbc.com/news/647721.

10. Zachary Coile, "Chilling 911 Call from Stricken Postal Worker; Frightened and Short of Breath, He Already Suspected Anthrax," *San Francisco Chronicle,* November 8, 2001, A1. Interagency communication gaps were indeed an issue. Caron Chess and Lee Clarke, "Facilitation of Risk Communication during the Anthrax Attacks of 2001: The Organizational Backstory," *American Journal of Public Health* 97, no. 9 (2007): 1578–83. The Postal Service's attribution of blame to the CDC would continue throughout the postmortem assessments, including, for example, in the GAO report *Better Guidance Is Needed to Ensure an Appropriate Response to Anthrax Contamination,* Report GAO-04-239 (Washington, D.C.: U.S. Government Accountability Office, 2004), esp. 4–5.

11. Ellen Gamerman, "Postal Employees Are Rankled; Workers Question Why Anthrax Case Did Not Close Office," *Baltimore Sun,* October 23, 2001, A1.

12. GAO, *Better Guidance Needed,* 32.

13. Gamerman, "Postal Employees Are Rankled." Even after the deaths of Morris and Curseen, postal officials were still telling postal workers that they should not worry unless they received a follow-up call. Frances Clines, "Being Left in the Gloom of Night over Threat," *New York Times,* October 22, 2001, B07.

14. Robert Schlesinger, "Fighting Terror the Anthrax Scare; DC Mayor Sees No Bias in Test Process," *Boston Globe,* October 25, 2001, A26.

15. Wiley A. Hall, "Urban Rhythms: Class Dictated Our Response to Anthrax," *Washington Afro-American,* November 19, 2001, 110, no. 12, A2. See also Hall, "Urban Rhythms: Terrorism Is Winning Its First Round of This War," *Baltimore Afro-American,* November 2, 2001, 110, no. 11, A2.

16. As of 2001, the Smithsonian Institution's web guide to African American resources at the museums specifically highlighted the National Postal Museum, pointing out that for years the Postal Service was the only federal agency that employed African Americans and that it remained the largest civilian employer of people of color. According to the Smithsonian, 21 percent of its more than 760,000 employees are African American. "African American Resources at the Smithsonian," http://www.si.edu/opa/afafam/npm.htm. According to Julianne Malveaux, while only 11 percent of the labor force is African American, 28 percent of postal workers are. Malveaux, "Race, Class, and Crass: Always Work at the Post Office," *Sun Reporter,* October 25, 2001, 58, no. 95, 6.

17. Frances Beal, "Race and Class Bias Infects Anthrax Fight," *Black World Today,* http://www.tbwt.com/views/feat/feat7051.asp.

18. E.g., Michael Goodin, "The Wrong Bodies Are on the Sacrificial Altar," *Michigan Chronicle,* November 13, 2001, 65, no. 6, A6; Bernice Powell Jackson, "Ode to Postal Workers," *Oakland Post,* December 5, 2001, 38, no. 49, 4; and Malveaux, "Race, Class, and Crass."

19. Ralph Wiley, "D.C. Talk," http://espn.go.com/page2/s/wiley-011025.

20. Blanchard et al., "In Their Own Words."

21. E.g., Marsha D. Lillie-Banton, Wilhelmina Leigh, and Ana Alfaro-Carera, *Achieving Equitable Access: Studies of Health Care Issues Affecting Hispanics and African Americans* (Washington, D.C.: Joint Center for Political and Economic Studies, 1996).

22. E.g., Clovis E. Semmes, *Racism, Health, and Post-Industrialism: A Theory of African-American Health* (Westport, Conn.: Praeger, 1996).

23. Hamil Harris, Jamie Stockwell, and Monte Reel, "Neighbors Remember 2 Postal Workers; Both Residents of Prince George's County," *Washington*

Post, October 25, 2001, T03. See also Martin Weil, "Anthrax Victims Extolled for Service to Neighborhoods," *Washington Post,* October 23, 2001, A10. More touching details of Curseen's middle-class life are from Lisa Simeone, *Weekend All Things Considered,* October 27, 2001. Curseen was even described by his mother as a "health freak" who "jogged around his neighborhood three mornings a week, downed eight glasses of water a day, and never even drank Communion wine." See Angie Cannon, "Unlikely Foot Soldiers in the War against Terror," *U.S. News and World Report,* November 5, 2001, 18.

24. Of Marquette University, in Wisconsin. Greg Garland, "Postal Service Anthrax Victims Are Mourned; One Brentwood Worker Active in Community, the Other 'Very Private,'" *Baltimore Sun,* October 24, 2001, 7A.

25. Thomas Frank and Ellen Yan, "America's Ordeal; a Tale of Two Capitols," *Newsday* [Long Island, NY], October 24, 2001, A04.

26. Amy Alexander, "Going Postal—for Good Reason," http://africana .com/. A shorter version of this article also appeared as Alexander, "Second-Class Postals," *Nation,* December 10, 2001, 6.

27. "Two New Anthrax Deaths Confirmed," *New York Beacon,* October 31, 2001, 8, no. 43, 2.

28. Indeed, at the time of the anthrax attacks, I did have some Cipro on hand left over from my recent trip to West Africa. I had taken several courses of Cipro over the years while traveling in South Asia, Latin America, and West Africa, with absolutely no medical supervision beyond the travel clinic's initial prescription.

29. Leslie Hausmann, Shasha Gao, Edward S. Lee, and C. Kent Kwoh, "Racial Disparities in the Monitoring of Patients on Chronic Opioid Therapy," *PAIN* 154, no. 1 (2013): 46–52.

30. Ana I. Balsa and Thomas G. McGuire, "Prejudice, Clinical Uncertainty and Stereotyping as Sources of Health Disparities," *Journal of Health Economics* 22, no. 1 (2003): 89–116.

31. Kirk Johnson, "The Victim; Demanding a Diagnosis, He Lives to Tell the Tale of Anthrax," *New York Times,* December 3, 2001, A1.

32. Editorial, "So-Called 'Little People' Get Left out of Loop," *Buffalo News,* October 29, 2001, B4.

33. Associated Press, November 8, 2001.

34. Avram Goldstein, "Mail Worker's Family Sues HMO over Death; Man's Anthrax Misdiagnosed as a Cold," *Washington Post,* November 14, 2001, B04.

35. Associated Press, November 8, 2001.

36. Luciana Borio, D. Frank, V. Mani, C. Chiriboga, M. Pollanen, M. Ripple, S. Ali et al., "Death due to Bioterrorism-Related Anthrax: Report of Two Patients," *JAMA* 286, no. 20 (2001): 2554–59.

37. Johnson, "The Victim."

38. Johnson.

39. *Washington Post,* "Lawsuit Over Anthrax Settled," August 9, 2002.

40. Goldstein, "Mail Worker's Family Sues HMO."

41. Goldstein.

42. Goldstein.

43. Goldstein.

44. T. M. Luhrmann, "Commentary," *Culture, Medicine, and Psychiatry* 25 (2001): 469.

45. Luhrmann.

46. Both of these historical precedents are cited by Alexander, "Going Postal."

47. Not long after this event, the Institute of Medicine released a study that controlled for insurance and found that attributing the racial differential to lack of access is incomplete. Given the same insurance, minorities receive less care. Sheryl Gay Stolberg, "Minorities Get Inferior Care, Even If Insured, Study Finds," *New York Times,* March 21, 2002, A1.

48. Frank and Yan, "America's Ordeal."

49. Steve Twomey and Justin Blum, "How the Experts Missed Anthrax; Brentwood Cases Defied Assumptions about Risks," *Washington Post,* November 19, 2001, A1.

50. This point about how compressed air machines work was one that employees raised in their criticism of the CDC and Postal Service response. GAO, *Better Guidance Is Needed,* 24.

51. Marie Coco, "We're All in This Together, but Actually We Aren't," *Newsday* [Long Island, NY], October 25, 2001, A44.

52. "So-Called 'Little People,'" B4. Kaiser reprised this line in the suit filed against it. "Mr. Morris lost his life because a criminal committed an unspeakable, cowardly act of terror. He died because someone put anthrax into an envelope, and sent it through the mail. We at Kaiser Permanente share the community's outrage at this senseless crime, and join in the hope that the perpetrator will be brought to justice." U.S. Newswire, "Kaiser Permanente Statement on Thomas L. Morris, Jr. Lawsuit," March 26, 2002.

53. The question of who perpetrated the attacks is beyond my scope, but feminist antiracist analysis can fruitfully be put there as well. See Gwen

D'Arcangelis, "Defending White Scientific Masculinity," *International Feminist Journal of Politics* 18, no. 1 (2016): 119–38.

54. Todd Purdum, "The Disease; More Checked for Anthrax; U.S. Officials Admit Underestimating Mail Risks," *New York Times,* October 25, 2001.

55. "So-Called 'Little People.'"

56. Schlesinger, "Fighting Terror."

57. Schlesinger.

58. Amy Alexander, "Bleaching the Disaster," http://africana.com/.

59. Unfortunately, I didn't have the capacity to do the necessary research to adequately review the television coverage, but in the print media, the distinction was stark. The U.S. sources of talk about race and this tragedy I found were on television-related sources MSNBC.com, ESPN.com, and Black-related sources Africana.com and *Black World Today.*

60. Toby Harnden, "Black Postal Workers Angered by Treatment Delay," *Daily Telegraph* [London], October 24, 2001, 11.

61. Among them, Gamerman, "Postal Employees Are Rankled"; "So-Called 'Little People'"; Coco, "We're All in This Together"; Frank and Yan, "America's Ordeal"; Eleanor Clift, "Capitol Letter: Bad PR: Is Anthrax Testing in Washington Elitist?," *Newsweek,* October 25, 2001. Except when noted, none of the articles I read mentioned that these victims were Black.

62. Twomey and Blum, "How the Experts Missed Anthrax."

63. *Washington Informer,* "No Time for Double Standards," October 31, 2001, 39, no. 2, 16.

64. Alexander, "Going Postal."

65. Borio et al., "Death due to Bioterrorism-Related Anthrax." The similar report on the survivors also left out mention of race, describing patient 1 as "a 56-year-old male postal worker" and patient 2 as "a 56-year-old man who worked at the Brentwood post office in the mail sorting facility." Thom A. Mayer, Susan Bersoff-Matcha, Cecele Murphy, James Earls, Scott Harper, Denis Pauze, Michael Nguyen et al., "Clinical Presentation of Inhalational Anthrax Following Bioterrorism Exposure: Report of 2 Surviving Patients," *JAMA* 286, no. 20 (2001): 2549–53.

66. For relevant discussion of the use of racial categories in medical research and practice, see Lundy Braun, Anne Fausto-Sterling, Duana Fullwiley, Evelynn M. Hammonds, Alondra Nelson, William Quivers, Susan M. Reverby, and Alexandra E. Shields, "Racial Categories in Medical Practice: How Useful Are They?," *PLoS Medicine* 4, no. 9 (2007): e271.

67. Robert S. Schwartz has compellingly argued that identifying inadequacy

of care should be the unique use of race as a concept in medicine. Schwartz, "Racial Profiling in Medical Research," *New England Journal of Medicine* 344, no. 18 (2001): 1392–93.

68. Veena Das, "Violence and Translation," *Anthropological Quarterly* 75, no. 1 (2001): 108.
69. Das, 109.
70. Nelson, "Façade of National Unity."

2. UN/NATURAL DISASTER

1. The timeline here comes from Will Drye, "Hurricane Katrina: The Essential Timeline," *National Geographic,* September 14, 2005, https://www.nationalgeographic.com/news/2005/9/weather-hurricane-katrina-timeline/.
2. "Hurricane Katrina," *New York Times,* September 25, 2012, https://www.nytimes.com/topic/subject/hurricane-katrina.
3. Many have made this point about the unnaturalness of the disaster, for example, Jeremy I. Levitt and Matthew C. Walker, *Hurricane Katrina: America's Unnatural Disaster* (Lincoln: University of Nebraska Press, 2009).
4. Robert Roos, "Hurricane Katrina Sparks Fears of Disease Outbreaks," Centers for Infectious Disease Research and Policy, September 2, 2005, http://www.cidrap.umn.edu/news-perspective/2005/09/hurricane-katrina-sparks-fears-disease-outbreaks.
5. Roos.
6. An early paper coming to this conclusion was P. Gregg Greenough and Thomas D. Kirsch, "Hurricane Katrina: Public Health Response— Assessing Needs," *New England Journal of Medicine* 355, no. 15 (2005): 1544–46.
7. Mary Alice Mills, Donald Edmonson, and Crystal L. Park, "Trauma and Stress Response among Hurricane Katrina Evacuees," *American Journal of Public Health* 97, Suppl. 1 (2007): S116–23. The authors note that the effect was particularly strong for Black evacuees. For discussion of both short-term and long-term impacts of psychosocial stress on cardiovascular disease among those impacted by Katrina, see also Carl J. Lavie, Thomas C. Gerber, and William L. Lanier, "Hurricane Katrina: The Infarcts beyond the Storm," *Disaster Medicine and Public Health Preparedness* 3, no. 3 (2009): 131–35.
8. Ninon A. Becquart, Elena N. Naumova, Gitanjali Singh, and Kenneth

K. H. Chui, "Cardiovascular Disease Hospitalizations in Louisiana Parishes' Elderly before, during and after Hurricane Katrina," *International Journal of Environmental Research and Public Health* 16, no. 1 (2019): 74.

9. Kevin U. Stephens et al., "Excess Mortality in the Aftermath of Hurricane Katrina: A Preliminary Report," *Disaster Medicine and Public Health Preparedness* 1, no. 1 (2007): 15–20, esp. 19.

10. Matthew N. Peters, John C. Moscona, Morgan J. Katz, Kevin B. Deandrade, Henry C. Quevedo, Sumit Tiwari, Andrew R. Burchett et al., "Natural Disasters and Myocardial Infarction: The Six Years after Hurricane Katrina," *Mayo Clinic Proceedings* 89, no. 4 (2014): 472–77; John C. Moscona, Matthew N. Peters, Rohit Maini, Paul Katigbak, Bradley Deere, Holly Gonzales, Christopher Westley et al., "The Incidence, Risk Factors, and Chronobiology of Acute Myocardial Infarction Ten Years after Hurricane Katrina," *Disaster Medicine and Public Health Preparedness* 13, no. 2 (2019): 217–22.

11. Sjaak van der Geest, Susan Reynolds White, and Anita Hardon, "The Anthropology of Pharmaceuticals: A Biographical Approach," *Annual Review of Anthropology* 25 (1996): 153–78.

12. Michel Foucault, *"Society Must Be Defended": Lectures at the Collège de France, 1975–6,* ed. Mauro Bertani and Alessandro Fontana, trans. David Macey (New York: Picador, 1997).

13. Joseph B. Treaster, "Superdome: Haven Quickly Becomes Ordeal," *New York Times,* September 1, 2005, http://www.nytimes.com/2005/09/01/us/nationalspecial/superdome-haven-quicklybecomes-an-ordeal.html.

14. American College of Cardiology annual meeting, New Orleans, La., March 24–27, 2007. I had attended many of these kinds of medical meetings in the years leading up to this one as part of the research for my first book, *Medicating Race: Heart Disease and Durable Preoccupations with Difference* (Durham, N.C.: Duke University Press, 2012).

15. There also is a resonance here with the broader racialized framing of suffering Black patients as "drug seeking," in which, for example, sickle cell patients seeking pain relief come to be seen as "a variant of the inner city drug addict stereotype." Keith Wailoo, *Dying in the City of the Blues: Sickle Cell Anemia and the Politics of Race and Health* (Chapel Hill: University of North Carolina Press, 2001), 23.

16. For a discussion of the turn-of-the-twentieth-century foundations of the racialization of the criminalization of drugs, with special attention to New Orleans and Atlanta, see Michael M. Cohen, "Jim Crow's Drug War: Race, Coca Cola, and the Southern Origins of Drug Prohibition," *Southern Cultures* 12, no. 3 (2006): 55–79. For discussion of broader

articulations of drugs as a threat that racialized groups pose to white suburban order, see Matthew D. Lassiter, "Impossible Criminals: The Suburban Imperatives of America's War on Drugs," *Journal of American History* 102, no. 1 (2015): 126–40, and Kane Race, "Drugs and Domesticity: Fencing the Nation," *Cultural Studies Review* 10, no. 2 (2004): 62–84.

17. Michelle Alexander, *The New Jim Crow: Mass Incarceration in the Age of Colorblindness* (New York: New Press, 2010).

18. See, e.g., Gail Garfield, "Hurricane Katrina: The Making of Unworthy Disaster Victims," *Journal of African American Studies* 10 (2007): 55–74.

19. Harris-Perry, *Sister Citizen*, 11.

20. Rebecca Solnit, "Reconstructing the Story of the Storm: Hurricane Katrina at Five," *Nation*, August 26, 2010.

21. Solnit.

22. Dan Berger, "Constructing Crime, Framing Disaster: Routines of Criminalization and Crisis in Hurricane Katrina," *Punishment and Society* 11, no. 4 (2009): 491–510.

23. Kathleen Tierney, Christine Bevc, and Erica Kuligowski, "Metaphors Matter: Disaster Myths, Media Frames, and Their Consequences in Hurricane Katrina," *Annals of the American Academy of Political and Social Science* 604, no. 1 (2006): 62.

24. Tierney et al., esp. 66.

25. Robin D. G. Kelley, "What Kind of Society Values Property over Black Lives?," *New York Times*, June 18, 2020.

26. Havidan Rodriguez, Joseph Trainor, and Enrico L. Quarantelli, "Rising to the Challenges of a Catastrophe: The Emergent and Prosocial Behavior Following Hurricane Katrina," *Annals of the American Academy of Political and Social Science* 604, no. 1 (2006): 82–101.

27. Agence France-Presse, "Troops Deployed in Anarchic New Orleans with Shoot to Kill Orders," September 2, 2005. This quote appeared, for example, in the *New York Times*: "The guardsmen were posted at major intersections, and Army vehicles patrolled the streets, seeking to quell the looting and unrestrained crime that has shocked the nation. Some 300 members of the Arkansas National Guard, just back from Iraq, were among those deployed from foreign assignments specifically to bring order. 'I have one message for these hoodlums,' said Gov. Kathleen Babineaux Blanco of Louisiana. 'These troops know how to shoot and kill, and they are more than willing to do so if necessary.'" James Dao and N. R. Kleinfield, "Conditions in New Orleans Still Dire—Pumping May Take Months," *New York Times*, September 3, 2005.

28. D'Ann R. Penner and Keith C. Ferdinand, *Overcoming Katrina: African*

American Voices from the Crescent City and Beyond (New York: Palgrave Macmillan, 2009), xix.

29. Louisa Edgerly, "Difference and Political Legitimacy: Speakers' Construction of 'Citizen' and 'Refugee' Personae in Talk about Hurricane Katrina," *Western Journal of Communication* 75, no. 3 (2011): 304–22.

30. Adeline Masquelier, "Why Katrina's Victims Aren't Refugees: Musings on a 'Dirty' Word," *American Anthropologist* 108, no. 4 (2006): 736.

31. For insightful reflection on contrasts in empathy toward differently racialized refugees and impoverished Black American patients, see Michelle Munyikwa, "Racialization, Affect, and Refuge," *Anthropology News* 58, no. 1 (2017): e226–29.

32. Linsey McGoey, Julian Reiss, and Ayo Wahlberg, "The Global Health Complex," *BioSocieties* 6, no. 1 (2011): 1–9. This connection between partial citizenship and racialization is one that links Katrina far more closely to Hurricane Maria, which devastated Puerto Rico in 2017, than with other damaging storms, such as 2012's Hurricane Sandy, which impacted a large swath of coastline including New York City.

33. Stephanie Strom, "After Storm, Relief Groups Consider More Work in U.S.," *New York Times,* January 1, 2006.

34. U.S. Congress, *Lessons Learned from Katrina in Public Health Care: Hearing before the Subcommittee on Bioterrorism and Public Health Preparedness of the Committee on Health, Education, Labor, and Pensions,* United States Senate, July 14, 2006, 6.

35. Andrea J. Sharma, Edward C. Weiss, Stacy L. Young, Kevin Stephens, Raoult Ratard, Susanne Straif-Bourgeois, Theresa M. Sokol, Peter Vranken, and Carol H. Rubin, "Chronic Disease and Related Conditions at Emergency Treatment Facilities in the New Orleans Area after Hurricane Katrina," *Disaster Medicine and Public Health Preparedness* 2, no. 1 (2008): 27–32.

36. Nancy Aldrich and William F. Benson, "Disaster Preparedness and the Chronic Disease Needs of Vulnerable Older Adults," *Preventing Chronic Disease* 5, no. 1 (2007): A27.

37. William E. Brown, "Surviving the Superdome," *JEMS: A Journal of Emergency Medical Services* 30, no. 11 (2005): 54–56.

38. Lydia Velazquez, Scott Dallas, Lisa Rose, Krista S. Evans, Rebecca Saville, Jialynn Wang, Sean K. Bradley, and James D. Bona, "A PHS Pharmacist Team's Response to Hurricane Katrina," *American Journal of Health-System Pharmacy* 63, no. 14 (2006): 1332–35, esp. 1333.

39. Marcello Tonelli, Natasha Wiebe, Brian Nadler, Ara Darzi, and Shahnawaz Rasheed, "Modifying the Interagency Emergency Health Kit to

Include Treatment for Non-communicable Diseases in Natural Disasters and Complex Emergencies," *BMJ Global Health* 1, no. 3 (2016): e000128.

40. Michael A. Jhung, Nadine Shehab, Cherise Rohr-Allegrini, Daniel A. Pollock, Roger Sanchez, Fernando Guerra, and Daniel B. Jernigan, "Chronic Disease and Disasters: Medication Demands of Hurricane Katrina Evacuees," *American Journal of Preventive Medicine* 33, no. 3 (2007): 207–10.

41. Eileen Koutnik-Fotopoulos, "In the Wake of Katrina, Chain Pharmacies and Drug Companies Join Forces," *Pharmacy Times,* October 1, 2005, http://www.pharmacytimes.com/publications/issue/2005/2005 -10/2005-10-9919. There are resonances with this PR and that in the Global South, as described by Stefan Ecks, "Global Pharmaceutical Markets and Corporate Citizenship: The Case of Novartis' Anti-cancer Drug Glivec," *BioSocieties* 3, no. 2 (2008): 165–81.

42. Martha I. Arrieta et al., "Providing Continuity of Care for Chronic Diseases in the Aftermath of Katrina: From Field Experience to Policy Recommendations," *Disaster Medicine Public Health Preparedness* 3, no. 3 (2009): 174–82.

43. This mapping of the terrain draws on Susan E. Bell and Anne E. Figert, "Medicalization and Pharmaceuticalization at the Intersections: Looking Backward, Sideways and Forward," *Social Science and Medicine* 75, no. 5 (2012): 775–83. A key text about pharmaceuticalization in the Global North would be Simon J. Williams, Paul Martin, and Jonathan Gabe, "The Pharmaceuticalisation of Society? A Framework for Analysis," *Sociology of Health and Illness* 33, no. 5 (2011): 710–25. A key text about pharmaceuticalization in the Global South would be João Biehl, "Pharmaceuticalization: AIDS Treatment and Global Health Politics," *Anthropological Quarterly* 80, no. 4 (2007): 1083–1126. The United States' famously unequal system has never fit in to the bifurcation easily, something that has become clearer since the economic crisis; see Anne Pollock, "Transforming the Critique of Big Pharma," *BioSocieties* 6, no. 1 (2011): 106–18.

44. See Anne Pollock and David S. Jones, "Coronary Artery Disease and the Contours of Pharmaceuticalization," *Social Science and Medicine* 131 (2015): 221–27.

45. Jeffrey W. Bethel, Sloane C. Burke, and Amber F. Britt, "Disparity in Disaster Preparedness between Racial/Ethnic Groups," *Disaster Health* 1, no. 2 (2013): 110–16.

46. See Jeremy A. Greene, *Prescribing by Numbers: Drugs and the Definition of Disease* (Baltimore: Johns Hopkins University Press, 2007); Joseph

Dumit, *Drugs for Life: How Pharmaceutical Companies Define Our Health* (Durham, N.C.: Duke University Press, 2012).

47. Earl S. Ford et al., "Chronic Disease in Health Emergencies: In the Eye of the Hurricane," *Preventing Chronic Disease* 3, no. 2 (2006): 3.

48. See, e.g., Stuart Galishoff, "Germs Know No Color Line: Black Health and Public Policy in Atlanta, 1900–1918," *Journal of the History of Medicine and Allied Sciences* 40, no. 1 (1985): 22–41. I have written about this association between whiteness/chronicity and Blackness/infectiousness in Pollock, *Medicating Race,* esp. in chapter 1, "Racial Preoccupations and Early Cardiology."

49. In international contexts, the racialization of infectious disease can be part of anti-Indigenous ideologies; see Charles L. Briggs and Clara Mantini-Briggs, *Stories in the Time of Cholera: Racial Profiling during a Medical Nightmare* (Berkeley: University of California Press, 2004).

50. See Priscilla Wald, "Imagined Immunities," in *Cultural Studies and Political Theory,* ed. Jodi Dean, 189–298 (Ithaca, N.Y.: Cornell University Press, 2000).

51. The false promise of pharmaceuticals as capable of alleviating marginalization is explored by Stefan Ecks, "Pharmaceutical Citizenship: Antidepressant Marketing and the Promise of Demarginalization in India," *Anthropology and Medicine* 12, no. 3 (2005): 239–54.

52. Ruth E. Berggren and Tyler J. Curiel, "After the Storm—Health Care Infrastructure in Post-Katrina New Orleans," *New England Journal of Medicine* 354, no. 15 (2006): 1550.

53. Rebecca B. Horn and Thomas D. Kirsch, "Disaster Response 2.0: Noncommunicable Disease Essential Needs Still Unmet," *American Journal of Public Health* 108 (2018): S202–3.

54. John E. Salvaggio, *New Orleans' Charity Hospital: A Story of Physicians, Politics and Poverty* (Baton Rouge: Louisiana State University Press, 1992).

55. K. Brad Ott, "Healthcare and Human Rights Consequences of the Closure of New Orleans' Charity Hospital after Hurricane Katrina," *Race, Gender, and Class* Supplement (2015): 160–83, https://search.proquestcom/docview/1749900978. Even as of this writing almost fifteen years later, the building complex remains abandoned.

56. M. Janine Brodie, Erin Weltzien, Drew Altman, Robert J. Blendon, and John M. Benson, "Experiences of Hurricane Katrina Evacuees in Houston Shelters: Implications for Future Planning," *American Journal of Public Health* 96, no. 8 (2006): 1402–8. Many other sources also highlight the detrimental impact of those dispersed by the storm lacking their

medical records, e.g., Crystal Franco, Eric Toner, Richard Waldhorn, Beth Maldin, Tara O'Toole, and Thomas V. Inglesby, "Systemic Collapse: Medical Care in the Aftermath of Hurricane Katrina," *Biosecurity and Bioterrorism: Biodefense Strategy, Practice, and Science* 4, no. 2 (2006): 135–46.

57. Ott, "Healthcare and Human Rights."

58. Jean Ait Belkhir and Christiane Charlemaine, "New Orleans' Katrina Recovery for Whom and What? A Race, Gender and Class Approach," *Race, Gender, and Class* Supplement (2015): 8–24, https://search.proquest.com/docview/1749901092.

59. Ronald C. Kessler and Hurricane Katrina Community Advisory Group, "Hurricane Katrina's Impact on the Care of Survivors with Chronic Medical Conditions," *Journal of General Internal Medicine* 22, no. 9 (2007): 1225–30.

60. Kessler.

61. Sandeep Gautam et al., "Effect of Hurricane Katrina on the Incidence of Acute Coronary Syndrome at a Primary Angioplasty Center in New Orleans," *Disaster Medicine and Public Health Preparedness* 3, no. 3 (2009): 144–50.

62. Peters et al., "Natural Disasters and Myocardial Infarction."

63. Moscona et al., "Incidence, Risk Factors, and Chronobiology."

64. Susan Cutter, "The Geography of Social Vulnerability: Race, Class, and Catastrophe," Social Sciences Research Council forum on "Understanding Katrina: Perspectives from the Social Sciences," https://items.ssrc.org/understanding-katrina/the-geography-of-social-vulnerability-race-class-and-catastrophe/.

65. These two phenomena are not completely disconnected: Anna Hartnell highlights that the "branding" of New Orleans as a "culturally backward 'museum,' as well as an excessive 'party town,' is a superficial aspect of the city's marginality," and yet these aspects combine with a "genuinely transgressive cultural legacy" rooted in the cultural practices of formerly enslaved people. Anna Hartnell, *After Katrina: Race, Neoliberalism, and the End of the American Century* (Albany, N.Y.: SUNY Press, 2017), 3.

66. David Atkins and Ernest M. Moy, "Left Behind: The Legacy of Hurricane Katrina," *British Medical Journal* 331 (2005): 916.

67. Atkins and Moy, 917.

68. Foucault, *"Society Must Be Defended."*

69. Foucault, 241.

70. Foucault, 245.

71. Foucault, 245.

72. Foucault, 254–60.

73. There is a robust body of scholarship that critiques Foucault's conceptualization of biopolitics on the basis of the centrality of Eurocentrism and racism to the Western conceptualization of the "human" itself that is beyond my scope but certainly worthy of exploration. Perhaps the most comprehensive is Alexander Weheliye, *Habeas Viscus: Racializing Assemblages, Biopolitics, and Black Feminist Theories of the Human* (Durham, N.C.: Duke University Press, 2014).

74. Sociologist Kathleen Tierney argued in her analysis of Katrina that "virtually nothing has been done since 9–11 to make this nation safer" and that "indeed, the opposite is the case." Tierney, "The Red Pill," Social Sciences Research Council forum on "Understanding Katrina: Perspectives from the Social Sciences,"https://items.ssrc.org/understanding-katrina/the-red-pill/.

75. Harris-Perry, *Sister Citizen*, 11.

3. MASS INCARCERATION

1. Bob Herbert, "For Two Sisters, the End of an Ordeal," *New York Times*, December 31, 2010; NAACP and Solitary Watch, Scott Sisters: Mississippi Justice, 2011, http://womenandprison.org/social-justice/view/help_free_the_scott_sisters/; Curtis Stephen, "Sisters Freed from Mississippi Jail," *Crisis*, Winter 2011, 33–35.

2. Christopher Burkle, "The Mississippi Decision Exchanging Parole for Kidney Donation: Is This the Beginning of Change for Altruistic-Based Human Organ Donation Policy in the United States?," *Mayo Clinic Proceedings* 86, no. 5 (2011): 414–18; Arthur Caplan, "The Use of Prisoners as a Source of Organs—an Ethically Dubious Practice," *American Journal of Bioethics* 11, no. 10 (2011): 1–5; Aviva Goldberg and Joel Frader, "Prisoners as Living Donors: The Case of the Scott Sisters," *American Journal of Bioethics* 11, no. 10 (2011): 15–16; Jennifer L. Visconti, "Exchanging a Kidney for Freedom: The Illegality of Conditioning Prison Releases on Organ Donations," *New England Journal of Criminal and Civil Confinement* 38 (2012): 199–217.

3. Criminal Trial Transcript, http://www.scribd.com/doc/35281862/Scott-transcript.

4. Bob Herbert, "So Utterly Inhumane," *New York Times*, October 12, 2010; Ward Schaefer, "Scott Sisters Appear Before the Parole Board," *Jackson Free Press*, December 15, 2010.

5. Schaefer, "Scott Sisters Appear."

6. Herbert, "So Utterly Inhumane."

7. Asha Bandele, "Their Fight for Freedom," *Essence,* November 2011, 142. This explicitly Christian articulation is in line with the history of a great deal of civil rights organizing—most famously the Reverend Dr. Martin Luther King Jr.

8. *Free the Scott Sisters* (blog), http://freethescottsisters.blogspot.com/; Stephen, "Sisters Freed from Mississippi Jail."

9. Artaymis Ma'at, "The Scott Sisters Prevail!" *Jackson Advocate,* March 29, 2012, 1B.

10. NAACP, "Criminal Justice: Restoring Justice to a Damaged System," *NAACP 2010 Annual Report,* 14.

11. Brandon King, "Building Power in a Frontline Community: The Cooperation Jackson Model," *Socialism and Democracy* 30, no. 2 (2016): 220; Akinyele Umoja, "Introduction: The Political Legacy of Chokwe Lumumba," *Black Scholar* 48 no. 2 (2018): 2.

12. "The Shocking Case of the Scott Sisters!" *Flyer* (blog), 2010, http://www.scribd.com/doc/34548313/Flyer-Back.

13. Ward Schaefer, "Barbour Suspends Scott Sisters' Sentences," *Jackson Free Press,* December 29, 2010.

14. "3/25 Day of Blogging for the Scott Sisters!" *Free the Scott Sisters* (blog), March 22, 2010, http://freethescottsisters.blogspot.com/2010/03/325 -day-of-blogging-for-scott-sisters.html. The call was picked up by many Black bloggers, first for March 18 and then for March 25; see, e.g., Jesse Muhammad, "A Day of Blogging for the Scott Sisters . . . Black Blogosphere Stand Up!" March 18, 2020, http://jessemuhammad .blogs.finalcall.com/2010/03/day-of-blogging-for-scott-sistersblack.html.

15. Ward Schaefer, "Scott Sisters Rally Draws Hundreds to Capital," *Jackson Free Press,* September 15, 2020.

16. Herbert, "So Utterly Inhumane."

17. Leonard Pitts, "Sisters May or May Not Be Guilty, but Mississippi Assuredly Is," *Seattle Times,* November 21, 2010.

18. "Governor Barbour's Statement Regarding Release of Scott Sisters," published in the *Jackson Free Press,* with an accompanying article: Ward Schaefer, "Barbour Suspends Scott Sisters' Sentences."

19. Jamila Jefferson-Jones, "The Exchange of Inmate Organs for Liberty: Diminishing the 'Yuck Factor' in the Bioethics Repugnance Debate," *Journal of Gender, Race, and Justice* 16 (2013): 121.

20. Goldberg and Frader, "Prisoners as Living Donors," 15.

21. Timothy Williams, "Jailed Sisters Are Released for Kidney Transplant," *New York Times*, January 8, 2011, A13.

22. Executive Orders 1046 and 1047, posted on *Free the Scott Sisters* (blog), at http://www.scribd.com/doc/47626550/Gladys-Scott-Gov-Orders.

23. Emily Wagster Pettus, "Pardon Unlikely for Sisters Awaiting Transplant," Associated Press, April 1, 2011, http://abcnews.go.com/US/wireStory?id=13268768; Elizabeth Crisp and Gary Pettus, "Released from Jail, Mississippi Sisters Still Seek Full Pardon," *USA Today*, April 1, 2011.

24. James Ridgeway, "The Scott Sisters' 'Debt to Society' and the New Jim Crow," *Mother Jones*, January 7, 2011, https://www.motherjones.com/crime-justice/2011/01/scott-sisters-debt-society-and-new-jim-crow/.

25. Artaymis Ma'at, "Florida Policeman Leaves Jamie Scott Stranded on Freeway," *Jackson Advocate*, March 29, 2012, 1B.

26. Holbrook Mohr, "Sisters Out for Kidney Donation Want to Be Pardoned in Miss," *Boston Globe*, January 13, 2012.

27. Jimmie E. Gates, "Freed Scott Sister Must Lose 120 lbs," *USA Today*, January 26, 2011.

28. Melissa Nelson Gabriel, "Still Fighting: Scott Sisters Find New Life in Pensacola after Prison, Heartbreak," *Pensacola News Journal*, July 23, 2018.

29. Harold Gater, "Scott Sisters, Who Got Life for Armed Robbery, Continue to Ask Gov. Bryant for Release," *Mississippi Clarion Ledger*, July 29, 2019.

30. Angela Davis, "From the Prison of Slavery to the Slavery of Prison: Frederick Douglas and the Convict Lease System," in *The Angela Y. Davis Reader*, ed. Joy James, 74–95 (Malden, Mass.: Blackwell, 1998); Douglas A. Blackmon, *Slavery by Another Name: The Re-enslavement of African Americans from the Civil War to World War II* (New York: Doubleday, 2008).

31. Davis, "From the Prison of Slavery."

32. Alice Thomas-Tisdale, "Scott Sisters Attend Meeting on Black Boys," *Jackson Advocate*, April 5, 2012, 1A, 14A.

33. "Scott Sisters Speak in Brooklyn!" Clips from Malcolm X Grassroots Movement and National Conference of Black Lawyers Forum featuring Jamie and Gladys Scott and panelists Chokwe Lumumba (legal counsel to the Scott sisters), Michael Tarif Warren (lawyer activist), Marc Lamont Hill (activist, author, scholar), Rukia Lumumba (activist), April R. Silver (activist, writer), and a moderator. Forum held on

April 23, 2011, and posted to YouTube, May 15, 2011, https://www
.youtube.com/watch?v=NJKlWT7X7wk.

34. See Anthony Ryan Hatch, *Silent Cells: The Secret Drugging of Captive America* (Minneapolis: University of Minnesota Press, 2019), 16.

35. Estelle v. Gamble, 429 U.S. 97 (1976).

36. Jessica Bakeman, "Barbour: Suspended Sentences for the Sick Saves Miss. Money," *Clarion Ledger,* February 5, 2012.

37. See Nicholas Freudenberg, "Adverse Effects of US Jail and Prison Policies on the Health and Well-Being of Women of Color," *American Journal of Public Health* 92, no. 12 (2002): 1895–99; Dora M. Dumont, Brad Brockmann, Samuel Dickman, Nicole Alexander, and Josiah D. Rich, "Public Health and the Epidemic of Incarceration," *Annual Review of Public Health* 33 (2012): 325–39.

38. American Public Health Association, *Policy Statement 9123: Social Practice of Mass Imprisonment,* 1991, https://www.apha.org/policies-and-advocacy /public-health-policy-statements/policy-database/2014/07/29/10/00/ social-practice-of-mass-imprisonment.

39. Christopher Wildeman and Emily A. Wang, "Mass Incarceration, Public Health, and Widening Inequality in the USA," *The Lancet* 389 (2017): 1464–74.

40. Dora Dumont, Scott A. Allen, Brad Brockmann, and Nicole E. Alexander, "Incarceration, Community Health, and Racial Disparities," *Journal of Health Care for the Poor and Underserved* 24 (2013): 78–88.

41. Wildeman and Wang, "Mass Incarceration," 1468. Moreover, longer incarceration has more deleterious effects postincarceration. Evelyn J. Patterson, "The Dose–Response of Time Served in Prison on Mortality: New York State, 1989–2003," *American Journal of Public Health* 103, no. 3 (2013): 523–28.

42. See Anthony Ryan Hatch, "Billions Served: Prison Food Regimes, Nutritional Punishment, and Gastronomical Resistance," in *Captivating Technology: Race, Carceral Technoscience, and Liberatory Imagination in Everyday Life,* ed. Ruha Benjamin, 67–84 (Durham, N.C.: Duke University Press, 2019).

43. Ann J. Russ, Janet K. Shim, and Sharon R. Kaufman, "'Is There Life on Dialysis?': Time and Ageing in a Clinically Sustained Existence," *Medical Anthropology* 24, no. 4 (2005): 297–324.

44. Sherine Hamdy, "When the State and Your Kidneys Fail: Political Etiologies in an Egyptian Dialysis Ward," *American Ethnologist* 35, no. 4 (2008): 563.

45. Ma'at, "Scott Sisters Prevail!"
46. Adriana Petryna, *Life Exposed: Biological Citizens after Chernobyl* (Princeton, N.J.: Princeton University Press, 2002), 5.
47. Petryna, 6.
48. Nikolas Rose and Carlos Novas, "Biological Citizenship," in *Global Assemblages: Technology, Politics, and Ethics as Anthropological Problems,* ed. Aihwa Ong and Stephen Collier (Oxford: Blackwell, 2005), 458.
49. Vinh-Kim Nguyen, *The Republic of Therapy: Triage and Sovereignty in West Africa's Time of AIDS* (Durham, N.C.: Duke University Press, 2010), 109.
50. Vinh-Kim Nguyen, "Antiretroviral Globalism, Biopolitics, and Therapeutic Citizenship," in Ong and Collier, *Global Assemblages,* 143.
51. Nguyen, *Republic of Therapy,* 176.
52. Nguyen, "Antiretroviral Globalism," 143.
53. Nguyen, *Republic of Therapy,* 109.
54. Nguyen, 108.
55. Alondra Nelson, *Body and Soul: The Black Panther Party and the Fight against Medical Discrimination* (Minneapolis: University of Minnesota Press, 2013), 168.
56. Nelson, 184.
57. Aditya Bharadwaj, "Biosociality and Biocrossings: Encounters with Assisted Conception and Embryonic Stem Cells in India," in *Biosocialities, Genetics and the Social Sciences: Making Biologies and Identities,* ed. Sahra Gibbon and Carlos Novas, 98–116 (London: Routledge, 2008).
58. Jessica Martucci, "Negotiating Exclusion: MSM, Identity, and Blood Policy in the Age of AIDS," *Social Studies of Science* 4, no. 2 (2010): 235.
59. Michelle Goodwin, *Black Markets: The Supply and Demand of Human Body Parts* (Cambridge: Cambridge University Press, 2006), xiii.
60. Goldberg and Frader, "Prisoners as Living Donors." This question has also been explored, including mention of the Scott sisters case, in Virginie Vallée Guignard and Marie-Chantal Fortin, "Emerging Ethical Challenges in Living Kidney Donation," *Current Transplantation Reports* 6, no. 2 (2019): 192–98, and in R. Bisi Adeyemo, "Don't Break My Heart, My Achy Breaky Heart: A Call for Legislation to Expressly Grant Inmates the Right to Donate Their Non-vital Organs," *Howard Law Journal* 60, no. 3 (2017): 781–816.
61. Catherine Waldby and Robert Mitchell, "Real-Time Demand: Information, Regeneration, and Organ Markets," in *Tissue Economies: Blood, Organs, and Cell Lines in Late Capitalism* (Durham, N.C.: Duke University

Press, 2006): 180; see also Nancy Scheper-Hughes, "The Ends of the Body: Commodity Fetishism and the Global Traffic in Organs," *SAIS Review* 22, no. 1 (2002): 61–80.

62. There has been significant anthropological attention to Islam and organ donation, including Hamdy, "When the State and Your Kidneys Fail," but surprisingly little to Christianity and organ donation. In her monumental exploration of organ donation in North America and Japan, anthropologist Margaret Lock gestures to how religiosity matters, referring at one point to "in America, land of Christianity," but her meditations upon Christianity are mostly about how early and medieval Christianity provides the historical roots for contemporary ideas about organ donation. Lock, *Twice Dead: Organ Transplants and the Reinvention of Death* (Berkeley: University of California Press, 2001), 154.

63. Rev. Jeremy Tobin, "Thoughts on the Scott Sisters: 'The Land Is Not Yet Free!'" *Jackson Advocate,* June 12, 2012.

64. This is not to deny that these categories and their relationship with state power, on one hand, and biomedical research, on the other, are tremendously problematic. See Steven Epstein, *Inclusion: The Politics of Difference in Medical Research* (Chicago: University of Chicago Press, 2007); Geoffery Bowker and Susan Leigh Star, *Sorting Things Out: Classification and Its Consequences* (Cambridge, Mass.: MIT Press, 1999); Ian Whitmarsh and David S. Jones, eds., *What's the Use of Race? Modern Governance and the Biology of Difference* (Cambridge, Mass.: MIT Press, 2010).

65. Jonathan Xavier Inda, "Materializing Hope: Racial Pharmaceuticals, Suffering Bodies, and Biological Citizenship," in *Corpus: An Interdisciplinary Reader on Bodies and Knowledge,* ed. Monica J. Casper and Paisley Currah, 61–80 (New York: Palgrave Macmillan 2011).

66. Dorothy Roberts, "Race and the New Biocitizen," in Whitmarsh and Jones, *What's the Use of Race?,* 259–76.

67. Emily Lee, "Trading Kidneys for Prison Time: When Two Contradictory Legal Traditions Intersect, Which One Has Right of Way?" *University of San Francisco Law Review* 43 (2009): 507–57.

68. Burkle, "Mississippi Decision."

69. Scott Vrecko, "Therapeutic Justice in Drug Courts: Crime, Punishment and Societies of Control," *Science as Culture* 2, no. 18 (2010): 217–32.

70. Lawrence Cohen, "Where It Hurts: Indian Material for an Ethics of Organ Donation," *Deadalus* 128, no. 4 (1999): 135–65.

71. Cohen, 152.

72. Krista L. Lentine, Mark A. Schnitzler, Huiling Xiao, Georges Saab,

Paolo R. Salvalaggio, David Axelrod, Connie L. Davis, Kevin C. Abbott, and Daniel C. Brennan, "Racial Variation in Medical Outcomes among Living Kidney Donors," *New England Journal of Medicine* 363 (2010): 724–32.

73. Gater, "Scott Sisters."

74. Susan Donaldson James, "Scott Sisters Kidney Donation Threatens Organ Transplant Laws," *ABC News*, 2010, http://abcnews.go.com/Health/scott-sisters-kidney-donation-threatens-organ-transplant-laws/story?id=12515616.

75. Caplan, "Use of Prisoners."

76. Karla Holloway, *Private Bodies, Public Texts: Race, Gender, and a Cultural Bioethics* (Durham, N.C.: Duke University Press, 2011).

77. Laura Mamo and Jennifer R. Fishman, "Why Justice? Introduction to the Special Issue on Entanglements of Science, Ethics, and Justice," *Science, Technology, and Human Values* 38, no. 2 (2013): 160.

78. K. Anthony Appiah, *Experiments in Ethics* (Cambridge, Mass.: Harvard University Press, 2010), 197–98.

79. Paul Farmer, *Pathologies of Power: Health, Human Rights, and the New War on the Poor* (Berkeley: University of California Press, 2003), 174.

80. Reverby, *Tuskegee's Truths.*

81. For the broader context of control of Black women's reproduction, see Dorothy Roberts, *Killing the Black Body: Race, Reproduction, and the Meaning of Liberty* (New York: Vintage, 1998). For more extended consideration of the inevitably coercive nature of sterilization in prisons in particular, see Rachel Roth and Sara L. Ainsworth, "If They Hand You a Paper, You Sign It: A Call to End the Sterilization of Women in Prison," *Hastings Women's Law Journal* 26, no. 1 (2015): 7–50.

82. Michel Foucault, *Discipline and Punish: The Birth of the Prison,* trans. Alan Sheridan (1975; repr., New York: Vintage Books, 1995).

83. Alexander, *New Jim Crow.*

84. Loïc Wacquant, "From Slavery to Mass Incarceration: Rethinking the 'Race Question' in the US," *New Left Review* 13 (2002): 55.

85. Wacquant, 54.

86. Ruha Benjamin, "Catching Our Breath: Critical Race STS and the Carceral Imagination," *Engaging Science, Technology, and Society* 2 (2016): 145–56; Benjamin, *Captivating Technology*; Nadine Ehlers and Shiloh Krupar, "When Treating Patients Like Criminals Makes Sense: Medical Hot Spotting, Race and Debt," in *Subprime Health: Debt and Race in U.S. Medicine,* ed. Nadine Ehlers and Leslie Hinkson, 31–53 (Minneapolis: University of Minnesota Press); Hatch, *Silent Cells.*

4. ENVIRONMENTAL RACISM

1. Mike Colias, "How GM Saved Itself from the Flint Water Crisis: Rusting Engine Blocks Flagged a Big Problem," *Automotive News,* January 31, 2016, http://www.autonews.com/article/20160131/OEM01/302019964/how-gm-saved-itself-from-flint-water-crisis.

2. Ron Fonger, "General Motors Shutting Off Flint River Water at Engine Plant over Corrosion Worries," *M Live,* October 13, 2014, http://www.mlive.com/news/flint/index.ssf/2014/10/general_motors_wont_use_flint.html.

3. Regulators consider fifteen parts per billion to merit amelioration, and even five parts per billion to be cause for concern. Ninety percent of Flint homes tested had lead levels above twenty-seven parts per billion. Christopher Ingraham, "This Is How Toxic Flint's Water Really Is," *Washington Post,* January 15, 2016.

4. Ashley Southall, "State of Emergency Declared over Man-Made Water Disaster in Michigan City," *New York Times,* January 17, 2016. The formal gubernatorial request for support from the federal government is a key step by which state and local authorities that are overwhelmed by a disaster can get access to federal resources.

5. For an overview of this issue and additional resources, see John R. Scully, "*CORROSION* Assigns 'Editor's Choice' Open Access to Key Papers Related to the Water Crisis in Flint, Michigan," *Corrosion* 72, no. 4 (2016): 451–53.

6. Mitch Smith, Julie Bosman, and Monica Davey, "Flint's Water Crisis Started 5 Years Ago. It's Not Over," *New York Times,* April 25, 2019.

7. Curt Guyette, "Flint and Expected Consequences," *Detroit Metro Times,* April 18, 2018; Steve Carmody, "5 Years after Flint's Crisis Began, Is the Water Safe?," NPR, April 25, 2019; Julie Bosman, "Michigan to Pay $600 Million to Victims of Flint Water Crisis," *New York Times,* August 19, 2020.

8. "Society Must Be Defended" is a key phrase from the philosopher Michel Foucault as he introduces the idea of biopolitics and is discussed at more length in chapter 2.

9. Isabel Wilkerson, *The Warmth of Other Suns: The Epic Story of America's Great Migration* (New York: Vintage, 2011), 10.

10. U.S. Census Briefs, "The Black Population 2010," C2010BR-06, September 2011, p. 15. Flint is featured as eighth in the list of a table of "Ten Places with the Highest Percentage of Blacks or African Americans: 2010." This figure is for "Black or African American alone." The figure

for "Black or African American alone or in combination" is slightly higher—59.5 percent.

11. Michael Moore, dir., *Roger and Me* (Dog Eat Dog Films, 1989). Scholarship about the deindustrialization of Flint has been in dialogue with Moore's film as well, notably Steven P. Dandaneau, *A Town Abandoned: Flint, Michigan, Confronts Deindustrialization* (Albany: SUNY Press, 1996).

12. For a classic and comprehensive account of the sit-down strike and its legacies, see Sidney Fine, *Sit-Down: The General Motors Strike of 1936–1937* (Ann Arbor: University of Michigan Press, 1969).

13. Detroit is the most high-profile case of the imposition of racialized emergency management across many of Michigan's Black-majority cities; see Mark Jay and Philip Conklin, *A People's History of Detroit* (Durham, N.C.: Duke University Press, 2020), esp. 44–47.

14. David Fasenfest and Theodore Pride, "Emergency Management in Michigan: Race, Class and the Limits of Liberal Democracy," *Critical Sociology* 42, no. 3 (2016): 332: "Since 2009, eight Michigan cities (Allen Park, Benton Harbor, Detroit, Ecorse, Flint, Hamtramck, Lincoln Park, and Pontiac) have operated, or continue to operate, under an Emergency Manager (EM) appointed by the state's governor. In total, according to the 2010 US Census . . . , these cities have a combined population of 955,843, representing just 9.7 percent of the state's total population. At the same time, the cities accounted for a total of 699,225 African-American residents, representing just under half (49.8%) of all of the African-American residents in the state of Michigan."

15. For a foundational introduction to this theme, see Jean-Paul Sartre, "Colonialism Is a System," originally given as a speech in 1956, in *Colonialism and Neocolonialism*, trans. Azzedine Haddour, Steve Brewer, and Terry McWilliams, 30–47 (New York: Routledge, 2001).

16. Darnell Earley, who is Black, and Gerald Ambrose, who is white, are the two former emergency managers who have faced criminal charges for their role in the Flint water crisis. Monica Davey and Mitch Smith, "2 Former Flint Emergency Managers Charged over Tainted Water," *New York Times,* December 20, 2016.

17. See Jason Stanley, "The Emergency Manager: Strategic Racism, Technocracy, and the Poisoning of Flint's Children," *Good Society* 25, no. 1 (2016): 1–45.

18. The financial risks were known in advance, as is clear from Caitlin Devitt, "Michigan Deal Finances Flint Breakaway from Detroit Water," *Bond Buyer,* March 26, 2014.

19. Peter J. Hammer, "The Flint Water Crisis, the Karegnondi Water Authority and Strategic–Structural Racism," *Critical Sociology* 45, no. 1 (2019): 103–19, esp. 111.

20. Hammer.

21. Leonard M. Fleming, "Flint Mayor, State Clash over Water Tax Liens," *Detroit News,* June 27, 2017.

22. In this sense, "care" is like what M'charek and Casartelli characterize as "forensic care." Amade M'charek and Sara Casartelli, "Identifying Dead Migrants: Forensic Care Work and Relational Citizenship," *Citizenship Studies* 23, no. 7 (2019): 739. The well-being of the residents of Flint did eventually become a site of care among a significant network of scientists and others, because of crucial activism on the part of residents—for an accessible overview, see Anna Clark, *The Poisoned City: Flint's Water Crisis and the American Urban Tragedy* (New York: Henry Holt, 2018).

23. As per the revisions of the emergency manager law passed in 2011. Stanley, "Emergency Manager."

24. Malini Ranganathan, "Thinking with Flint: Racial Liberalism and the Roots of an American Water Tragedy," *Capitalism, Nature, Socialism* 27, no. 3 (2016): 17–33, esp. 27.

25. Stanley, "Emergency Manager."

26. Katie Levy, dir., *Here's to Flint* (ACLU of Michigan Documentary, 2016). The same activist statement is also quoted by Stanley and Pulido.

27. Yvette Shields, "Flint Will Stick with Great Lakes Authority Water, While Honoring Karegnondi Debt," *Bond Buyer,* April 19, 2017. Socializing the risk of the financial decisions made to benefit the few is another way in which the Flint experience resonates with structural adjustment, since holding the state responsible for decisions made by and for a few rulers is a key element of neocolonial fiscal governance—see, e.g., Noam Chomsky, "The Capitalist 'Principle' and Third World Debt," *Green Left Weekly,* May 24, 2000, https://www.greenleft.org.au/content/noam-chomsky-capitalist-principle-and-third-world-debt.

28. See Jenna M. Loyd, "Obamacare and Sovereign Debt," in *Subprime Health: Debt and Race in U.S. Medicine,* ed. Nadine Ehlers and Leslie R. Hinkson, 55–82 (Minneapolis: University of Minnesota Press, 2017).

29. See Stanley, "Emergency Manager," esp. 36–37.

30. Jones, "Levels of Racism," 1212.

31. Sociologist Peter J. Hammer terms the ability of emergency managers to profit from the public purse while disregarding the needs of the disempowered citizens *strategic racism,* which is to say "the manipulation of intentional racism, structural racism and unconscious biases for

economic or political gain, regardless of whether the actor has express racist intent." Hammer, "Flint Water Crisis," 104.

32. Jones, "Levels of Racism," 1212.

33. Laura Pulido, "Flint, Environmental Racism, and Racial Capitalism," *Capitalism Nature Socialism* 27, no. 3 (2016): 1–16.

34. For a good introduction to the ideologically laden moral logics of structural adjustment in Africa, see James Ferguson, "Demoralizing Economies: African Socialism, Scientific Capitalism, and the Moral Politics of Structural Adjustment," in his book *Global Shadows: Africa in the Neoliberal World Order,* 69–88 (Durham, N.C.: Duke University Press, 2006).

35. Jorge Furtado, dir., *Island of Flowers* (Casa de Cinema de Porto Alegre, 1989).

36. For a feminist critical race analysis of the problems of techno-utopic narratives, see Neda Atanasoski and Kalindi Vora, "Surrogate Humanity: Posthuman Networks and the (Racialized) Obsolescence of Labor," *Catalyst: Feminism, Theory, Technoscience* 1, no. 1 (2015).

37. Paul Egan, "Flint Red Flag: 2015 Report Urged Corrosion Control," *Detroit Free Press,* January 21, 2016, https://www.freep.com/story/news /local/michigan/flint-water-crisis/2016/01/21/flint-red-flag-2015-report -urged-corrosion-control/79119240/.

38. See Chelsea Grimmer, "Racial Microbiopolitics: Flint Lead Poisoning, Detroit Water Shut Offs, and the 'Matter' of Enfleshment," *Comparatist* 41 (2017): 19–40, esp. 25–26.

39. Janine MacLeod, "Water and the Material Imagination: Reading the Sea of Memory against the Flows of Capital," in *Thinking with Water,* ed. Celia Chen, Janine MacLeod, and Astrida Neimanis, 40–60 (Montreal: McGill-Queen's University Press, 2013), e.g., "Watery language naturalizes the movements of capital. To the degree that it is carried by aqueous imagery, capital is figured as a necessity, no less a biospheric feature than an ocean or a raincloud" (42), and later, "as investment comes to be regarded as an essential source of health, good livelihood, and agency, water's more fundamental association with these qualities falls into the background" (44).

40. Cecilia Chen, Janine MacLeod, and Astrida Neimanis, "Introduction: Toward a Hydrological Turn?" in Chen et al., *Thinking with Water,* 3.

41. Quoted in Pulido, "Flint, Environmental Racism, and Racial Capitalism," 11.

42. Marc de Leeuw and Sonja van Wichelen, "Legal Personhood in Postgenomic Times: Plasticity, Rights, and Relationality," in *Personhood in the*

Age of Biolegality: Brave New Law, ed. Marc van Leeuw and Sonja van Wichelen (Cham, Switzerland: Palgrave Macmillan, 2020), 60.

43. John Wisely, "Flint Residents Paid America's Highest Water Rates," *Detroit Free Press,* February 16, 2016, https://www.freep.com/ story/news/local/michigan/flint-water-crisis/2016/02/16/study-flint -paid-highest-rate-us-water/80461288/.

44. Andrew R. Highsmith, *Demolition Means Progress: Flint, Michigan, and the Fate of the American Metropolis* (Chicago: University of Chicago Press, 2015), esp. chapters 4 and 5, "Suburban Renewal" and "The Metropolitan Moment" (103–45). For discussion, see Michigan Civil Rights Commission, *The Flint Water Crisis: Systemic Racism through the Lens of Flint* (Lansing: Michigan Civil Rights Commission, February 17, 2017), 49–51.

45. Nikhil Anand, *Hydraulic City: Water and the Infrastructures of Citizenship in Mumbai* (Durham, N.C.: Duke University Press, 2017), 8.

46. See, e.g., K. Ravi Raman, "Community–Coca-Cola Interface: Political-Anthropological Concerns on Corporate Social Responsibility," *Social Analysis* 51, no. 3 (2007): 103–20.

47. See, e.g., Antina von Schnitzler, *Democracy's Infrastructure: Techno-politics and Protest after Apartheid* (Princeton, N.J.: Princeton University Press, 2016).

48. Astrida Neimanis, "Alongside the Right to Water, a Posthumanist Feminist Imaginary," *Journal of Human Rights and the Environment* 5, no. 1 (2014): 5–24, esp. 8.

49. Michelle Murphy, "Distributed Reproduction, Chemical Violence, and Latency," *Scholar and Feminist Online* 11, no. 3 (2013), https://sfonline.barnard.edu/life-un-ltd-feminism-bioscience-race/ distributed-reproduction-chemical-violence-and-latency/.

50. The tendency toward mysticism is even more striking in the field of "discard studies," which emphasizes the unpredictable liveliness of waste, often obscuring the brutal workings of power relations that create that unknowability; see Gabrielle Hecht, "Interscalar Vehicles for an African Anthropocene: On Waste, Temporality, and Violence," *Cultural Anthropology* 33, no. 1 (2018): 112.

51. Jane Bennett, *Vibrant Matter: A Political Ecology of Things* (Durham, N.C.: Duke University Press, 2010).

52. For an overview of this issue and additional resources, see Scully, "*CORROSION.*"

53. Monica Davey, "As Aid Floods into Flint, a Fix Remains Far Off," *New York Times,* March 6, 2016.

54. Paul Farmer is the most influential example, and he has discussed the concept this way: "The first notion is the preferential option for the poor. Any serious examination of epidemic disease has always shown that microbes also make a preferential option for the poor. But medicine and its practitioners, even in public health, do so all too rarely. Imagine how much unnecessary suffering we might collectively avert if our health care and educational systems, foundations, and nongovernmental organizations genuinely made a preferential option for the poor?" Farmer, "How Liberation Theology Can Inform Public Health," *Sojourners,* January 2014, https://sojo.net/magazine/january-2014/sacred-medicine. Politics of vulnerability is certainly fraught: Michigan is an epicenter of anti-abortion politics, in which claims of protecting vulnerable fetuses are used to justify controlling women. However, in Flint Lives Matter, the politics is one that prioritizes not a mystification of the unborn but the very concrete already here.

55. "Positive signs in the contemporary world are the growing awareness of the solidarity of the poor among themselves, their efforts to support one another, and their public demonstrations on the social scene which, without recourse to violence, present their own needs and rights in the face of the inefficiency or corruption of public authorities. By virtue of her own evangelical duty the Church feels called to take her stand beside the poor, to discern the justice of their requests, and to help satisfy them, without losing sight of the good of groups in the context of the common good." *Sollicitudo Rei Socialis,* para. 39.

56. Rob Nixon, *Slow Violence and the Environmentalism of the Poor* (Cambridge, Mass.: Harvard University Press, 2011), 2.

5. POLICE BRUTALITY

1. Foucault, *History of Sexuality Volume 1,* 138.
2. Abigail A. Sewell and Kevin A. Jefferson, "Collateral Damage: The Health Effects of Invasive Police Encounters in New York City," *Journal of Urban Health* 93, no. 1 (2016): 42–67.
3. As a classic analyst of theories of technological politics, Langdon Winner, canonically argued, "Its [technological politics's] starting point is a decision to take technical artifacts seriously. Rather than insist that we immediately reduce everything to the interplay of social forces, the theory of technological politics suggests that we pay attention to the characteristics of technical objects and the meaning of those characteristics."

Winner, "Do Artefacts Have Politics?" in *The Whale and the Reactor: A Search for Limits in an Age of High Technology* (Chicago: University of Chicago Press, 1986), 21–22.

4. This is most elaborated in terms of *sousveillance*, which is to say the surveilled observing the surveilling authorities from below, in a way that anticipates the use of smartphones to record police violence. Steve Mann, Jason Nolan, and Barry Wellman, "Sousveillance: Inventing and Using Wearable Computing Devices for Data Collection in Surveillance Environments," *Surveillance and Society* 1, no. 3 (2003): 331–55.

5. Carol Cole-Frowe and Richard Fausset, "Jarring Image of Police's Use of Force at Texas Pool Party," *New York Times,* June 8, 2015.

6. http://shine.forharriet.com/2015/06/19-year-old-woman-attacked-at -mckinney.html.

7. Brittney Cooper, "America's War on Black Girls: Why McKinney Police Violence Isn't about 'One Bad Apple,'" *Salon,* June 11, 2015, https:// www.salon.com/2015/06/10/americas_war_on_black_girls_why_ mckinney_police_violence_isnt_about_one_bad_apple/.

8. Mitch Mitchell, "Family Sues Ex-McKinney Officer for $5 Million for Excessive Force at Pool Party," *Fort Worth Star-Telegram,* January 3, 2017, https://www.star-telegram.com/news/local/community/dallas/ article124409854.html.

9. Alicia Garza, "A Herstory of the #BlackLivesMatter Movement," in *Are All the Women Still White? Rethinking Race, Expanding Feminisms,* ed. Janell Hobson, 23–28 (Albany, N.Y.: SUNY Press, 2016). For a compelling overview of the broader context of the emergence of Black Lives Matter, see Keeanga-Yamahtta Taylor, *From #BlackLivesMatter to Black Liberation* (Chicago: Haymarket Books, 2016).

10. Jane Margolis, with Rachel Estrella, Joanna Goode, Jennifer Jellison Holme, and Kim Nao, *Stuck in the Shallow End: Education, Race, and Computing* (Cambridge, Mass.: MIT Press, 2008).

11. Margolis et al., 24.

12. Jeff Wiltse, *Contested Waters: A Social History of Swimming Pools in America* (Chapel Hill: University of North Carolina Press, 2007), 1.

13. Wiltse, 2. Pools as prominent sites of segregation and civil rights activism are not exclusive to the U.S. context but has a fascinating history in many places, especially in other settler colonies. See, e.g., Penelope Edmonds, "Unofficial Apartheid, Convention and Country Towns: Reflections on Australian History and the New South Wales Freedom Rides of 1965," *Postcolonial Studies* 15, no. 2 (2012): 167–90.

14. Victoria W. Wolcott, *Race, Riots, and Roller Coasters: The Struggle over*

Segregated Recreation in America (Philadelphia: University of Pennsylvania Press, 2014).

15. Olga Khazan, "After the Police Brutality Video Goes Viral," *Atlantic,* July 29, 2019, https://www.theatlantic.com/politics/archive/2018/07/after-the-police-brutality-video-goes-viral/564863/.

16. "Best Places to Live: #1. McKinney, Texas," *Money,* September 19, 2014, http://money.com/money/collection-post/3312309/mckinney-texas-best-places-to-live/.

17. U.S. Census Bureau, QuickFacts, McKinney, Texas, https://www.census.gov/quickfacts/fact/table/mckinneycitytexas/POP060210.

18. Khazan, "After the Police Brutality Video."

19. Chun, "Race and/as Technology," 46.

20. Grace Elizabeth Hale, *Making Whiteness: The Culture of Segregation in the South, 1890–1940* (1998; repr., New York: Vintage, 2010).

21. Jon Schuppe and Craig Stanley, "McKinney Community Fights Charges of Racism Brought on by Pool Party Video," *NBC News,* June 8, 2015.

22. Naomi Adiv, "Hardening Racial Lines in Public Space: A Comment on the McKinney Pool Episode," *Metropolitics,* July 7, 2015, https://www.metropolitiques.eu/Hardening-Racial-Lines-in-Public.html.

23. Barbara Harris Combs, "A Jim Crow State of Mind: The Racialization of Space in the McKinney, Texas Pool Party Incident," *American Behavioral Scientist,* online first, June 30, 2019, https://doi.org/10.1177/0002764219859617.

24. Wiltse, *Contested Waters,* 124. See also Caleb P. Smith, "Reflections in the Water: Society and Recreational Facilities, a Case Study of Public Swimming Pools in Mississippi," *Southeastern Geographer* 52, no. 1 (2012): 39–54.

25. This is ubiquitous, albeit most obvious in high-profile venues such as the "swimsuit issue" of *Sports Illustrated.* See Laurel R. Davis, *The Swimsuit Issue and Sport: Hegemonic Masculinity in Sports Illustrated* (Albany, N.Y.: SUNY Press, 1997).

26. Matthew Haag and Cara Buckley, "Miss America Ends Swimsuit Competition, Aiming to Evolve in 'This Cultural Revolution,'" *New York Times,* June 5, 2018. For background, see Grace Slapak, "Sink or Swim: Deciding the Fate of the Miss America Swimsuit Competition," *Women Leading Change: Case Studies on Women, Gender, and Feminism* 4, no. 1 (2019): 72–92.

27. For example, London has banned body-shaming ads featuring bikini-clad women on the Tube. Jasper Jackson, "Sadiq Khan Moves to Ban Body-Shaming Ads from London Transport," *Guardian,* June 13, 2016.

28. Julia Thylin, "The Burkini as a Symbolic Threat: Anthropological Perspectives on the Ban of the Burkini on French Beaches 2016," master's thesis, Lund University, 2016.
29. Tanisha C. Ford, "A Black Girl Song for Dajerria," *QED: A Journal in GLBTQ Worldmaking* 4, no. 3 (2017): 156–60.
30. Ford, 158.
31. Ford, 158.
32. Ford, 157.
33. Sikivu Hutchinson, "Police Criminals and the Brutalization of Black Girls," *LA Progressive,* June 9, 2015, https://www.laprogressive.com/brutalization-of-black-girls/.
34. Ruth Nicole Brown, *Hear Our Truths: The Creative Potential of Black Girls* (Urbana: University of Illinois Press, 2013), 2.
35. Tom Dart and Amanda Holpuch, "Texas Pool Party Incident: Teen in Video Says Officer Was Provoked by 'Rudeness,'" *Guardian,* June 8, 2015, https://www.theguardian.com/us-news/2015/jun/08/texas-pool-party-police-dajerria-becton-eric-casebolt-rude.
36. Cooper, "America's War on Black Girls."
37. Nnennaya Amuchie, "'The Forgotten Victims': How Racialized Gender Stereotypes Lead to Police Violence against Black Women and Girls: Incorporating an Analysis of Police Violence into Feminist Jurisprudence and Community Activism," *Seattle Journal for Social Justice* 14, no. 3 (2016): 660.
38. See Jamelle Bouie, "Michael Brown Wasn't a Superhuman Demon, but Darren Wilson's Racial Prejudice Told Him Otherwise," *Slate News,* November 26, 2014, https://slate.com/news-and-politics/2014/11/darren-wilsons-racial-portrayal-of-michael-brown-as-a-superhuman-demon-the-ferguson-police-officers-account-is-a-common-projection-of-racial-fears.html; Erica Campbell, "Officer Wilson's Racialization of Mike Brown: A Discourse of Race, Gender, and Mental Health," *Journal of Gender Studies* 29, no. 2 (2020): 227–33. The full transcript of the police officer's aggrandizing testimony to the grand jury is publicly available: *State of Missouri v. Darren Wilson,* September 16, 2014, https://www.documentcloud.org/documents/1370569-grand-jury-volume-5.html#document/p216/a189399.
39. The McKinney pool party incident is invoked in the opening of the important book on the ways in which the "school-to-prison pipeline" critique must be expanded to include recognition of the harms to girls. Monique W. Morris, *Pushout: The Criminalization of Black Girls in Schools* (New York: New Press, 2016), 1–2. See also Kimberlé Williams Crenshaw,

with Priscilla Ocen and Jyoti Nanda, *Black Girls Matter: Pushed Out, Overpoliced and Underprotected* (New York: African American Policy Forum, 2015).

40. Chun, "Race and/as Technology," 57.

41. Benjamin, *Captivating Technology*, 1.

42. "Assault Swim," *The Daily Show,* June 8, 2015, YouTube video, https://www.youtube.com/watch?v=HbSBZycnyac.

43. Lalo Alcaraz, *Coming Soon: Attack of the 14-Year-Old Black Girl!,* June 10, 2015, http://www.pocho.com/coming-soon-attack-of-the-14-year-old-black-girl/.

44. Cartoon by Markus Prime. Featured in Andrea J. Ritchie, "Dajerria Becton Survived a Violent Arrest at a Pool Party and Went Viral," *Teen Vogue,* June 19, 2018, https://www.teenvogue.com/story/dajerria-becton-arrest-pool-party-viral. Although I was not able to reach the artist to secure permission to reprint the cartoon, I recommend that readers seek it out.

45. George E. Curry, "Fox News and AP Also Abused Black Youth," *North Dallas Gazette,* June 16, 2015, https://northdallasgazette.com/2015/06/16/fox-news-and-ap-also-abused-black-youth/.

46. For discussion of intersectionality in the broader social movement, see Melissa Brown, Rashawn Ray, Ed Summers, and Neil Fraistat, "#Say-HerName: A Case Study of Intersectional Social Media Activism," *Ethnic and Racial Studies* 40, no. 11 (2017): 1831–46.

47. Sherri Williams, "#SayHerName: Using Digital Activism to Document Violence against Black Women," *Feminist Media Studies* 16, no. 5 (2016): 922–25.

48. Armond R. Towns, "Geographies of Pain: #SayHerName and the Fear of Black Women's Mobility," *Women's Studies in Communication* 39, no. 2 (2016): 122–26.

49. For a rich exploration of the complex generativity of Black Twitter, see André Brock, *Distributed Blackness: African American Cybercultures* (New York: NYU Press, 2020).

50. One thoughtful article that invokes the Becton case among many others to make this case is I. Bennett Capers, "Race, Policing, and Technology," *North Carolina Law Review* 95, no. 4 (2017): 1241–92.

51. Benjamin, *Captivating Technology*, 3. See also Benjamin, *Race after Technology.*

52. Beth Coleman, "Race as Technology," *Camera Obscura: Feminism, Culture, and Media Studies* 24, no. 1 (2009): 177–207; Chun, "Race and/as Technology."

53. Chun, "Race and/as Technology," 38.
54. Chun, 56–57.
55. Coleman, "Race as Technology," 183.
56. Coleman.
57. This is the subject of a large body of scholarship. For a rich intersectional feminist account of how marginalized groups use Twitter to advance counternarratives and build activist networks, see Sarah J. Jackson, Moya Bailey, and Brooke Foucault Welles, #HashtagActivism: Networks of Race and Gender Justice (Cambridge, Mass.: MIT Press, 2020).
58. Coleman, "Race as Technology," 199.
59. Chun, "Race and/as Technology," 56–57.
60. Alondra Nelson edited a landmark special issue of the cultural studies journal Social Text on the topic of Afrofuturism, and her introduction provides a good route into the topic. Nelson, "Introduction: Future Texts," Social Text 20, no. 2 (2002): 1–15. See also Ruha Benjamin, "Introduction: Discriminatory Design, Liberating Imagination," in Benjamin, Captivating Technology, 1–24.
61. This is a prominent element, for example, of critique of race-based pharmaceuticals—e.g., Jonathan Kahn, who points out that health disparities are "caused by social discrimination and economic inequality" and argues that "the problem with marketing race-specific drugs is that it becomes easier to ignore the social realities and focus on the molecules." Kahn, Race in a Bottle, 194.

6. REPRODUCTIVE INJUSTICE

1. Her full name is "Alexis Olympia Ohanian Jr.," but her family calls her "Olympia."
2. Rob Haskell, "Serena Williams on Motherhood, Marriage, and Making Her Comeback," Vogue, January 10, 2018, https://www.vogue.com/article/serena-williams-vogue-cover-interview-february-2018.
3. Haskell.
4. Being Serena, season 1, episode 2, 9:20.
5. Serena Williams, Facebook, January 15, 2018, https://www.facebook.com/SerenaWilliams/videos/10156086135726834/.
6. African American women's mortality rate in childbirth is 42.8 per hundred thousand live births, compared with white women's mortality rate of 11 per hundred thousand live births. Emily E. Petersen, Nicole L. Davis, David Goodman, Shanna Cox, Nikki Mayes, Emily Johnston,

Carla Syverson et al., "Vital Signs: Pregnancy-Related Deaths, United States, 2011–2015, and Strategies for Prevention, 13 States, 2013–2017," *Morbidity Mortality Weekly Report* 68 (2019): 423–29.

7. Lindsay Schallon, "Serena Williams on the Pressure of Motherhood: 'I'm Not Always Going to Win,'" *Glamour,* April 27, 2018, https://www.glamour.com/story/serena-williams-motherhood-activism-me-too.

8. A recent biography has appropriately characterized Serena Williams as a "Digital Age Activist," giving that title to chapter 5 of Merlisa Lawrence Corbett, *Serena Williams: Tennis Champion, Sports Legend, and Cultural Heroine* (New York: Rowman and Littlefield, 2020).

9. For discussion of connections between Serena Williams's individual story and the data about Black women's maternal mortality, see Catherine D'Ignazio and Lauren F. Klein, *Data Feminism* (Cambridge, Mass.: MIT Press, 2020), 21–24.

10. For a useful primer on reproductive justice, see Loretta Ross and Rickie Solinger, *Reproductive Justice: An Introduction* (Oakland: University of California Press, 2017).

11. Dorothy Roberts, *Killing the Black Body: Race, Reproduction, and the Meaning of Liberty* (New York: Random House, 1997). A particularly powerful articulation of this key argument from the book as a whole comes on pp. 300–301.

12. SisterSong Women of Color Reproductive Justice Collective, "Reproductive Justice," https://www.sistersong.net/reproductive-justice.

13. SisterSong initiated the Trust Black Women project in response to antichoice billboards put up in Atlanta in 2010 that egregiously equated abortion among Black women with genocide, and the partnership has grown and developed since, in solidarity with Black Lives Matter. See https://trustblackwomen.org/our-roots.

14. More information about these groups can be found at Race/Biomed, http://www.racebiomed.org/, and Black Feminist Think Tank, http://www.sheriemrandolph.com/projects.

15. "Race, Biomedicine, Reproductive Justice: A Public Dialogue with Dr. Loretta Ross and Dr. Whitney Robinson," video, March 29, 2018, https://smartech.gatech.edu/handle/1853/59546. The question discussed comes at 1:23.

16. Dána-Ain Davis, *Reproductive Injustice: Racism, Pregnancy, and Premature Birth* (New York: NYU Press, 2019), 206.

17. Tressie McMillan Cottom, "Presumed Incompetent," in *Thick: And Other Essays,* 86 (New York: New Press, 2019).

18. Cottom.

19. Pain is probably the topic about which there is the most robust literature on doctors' reluctance to take women's complaints seriously; see Anke Samulowitz, Ida Gremyr, Erik Eriksson, and Gunnel Hensing, "'Brave Men' and 'Emotional Women': A Theory-Guided Literature Review on Gender Bias in Health Care and Gendered Norms towards Patients with Chronic Pain," *Pain Research and Management* (2018), https://doi.org/10.1155/2018/6358624.

20. Andreea A. Creanga, Cynthia J. Berg, Jean Y. Ko, Sherry L. Farr, Van T. Tong, F. Carol Bruce, and William M. Callaghan, "Maternal Mortality and Morbidity in the United States: Where Are We Now?," *Journal of Women's Health* 23, no. 1 (2014): 4. See also Judette M. Louis, M. Kathryn Menard, and Rebekah E. Gee, "Racial and Ethnic Disparities in Maternal Morbidity and Mortality," *Obstetrics and Gynecology* 125, no. 3 (2015): 690–94.

21. See, e.g., New York City Department of Health and Mental Hygiene, *Severe Maternal Morbidity in New York City, 2008–2012* (New York: New York City Department of Health and Mental Hygiene, 2016), 15.

22. Amy Roeder, "America Is Failing Its Black Mothers," *Harvard Public Health,* Winter 2019, 1–28.

23. For a concise overview of the weathering hypothesis, see Arline T. Geronimus, "Black/White Differences in the Relationship of Maternal Age to Birthweight: A Population-Based Test of the Weathering Hypothesis," *Social Science and Medicine* 42, no. 4 (1996): 589–97. Stress has also been implicated as a cause for high rates of premature birth among African American women; see, e.g., Carol J. Rowland Hogue and J. Douglas Bremner, "Stress Model for Research into Preterm Delivery among Black Women," *American Journal of Obstetrics and Gynecology* 192, no. 5 (2005): S47–55.

24. Christina Sharpe, *In the Wake: On Blackness and Being* (Durham, N.C.: Duke University Press, 2016), 104.

25. Roeder, "America Is Failing Its Black Mothers."

26. The idea of "accumulated insults" of living in a racist society comes from Nancy Krieger and "inaction in the face of need" from Camara Jones. Krieger, "Embodying Inequality: A Review of Concepts, Measures, and Methods for Studying Health Consequences of Discrimination," *International Journal of Health Services* 29, no. 2 (1999): 296; Jones, "Levels of Racism," 1212.

27. Khiara M. Bridges, *Reproducing Race: An Ethnography of Pregnancy as a Site of Racialization* (Berkeley: University of California Press, 2011), 112.

28. Bridges, 113.

29. California Newsreel with Vital Pictures, *Unnatural Causes: Is Inequality Making us Sick?*, episode 2, "When the Bough Breaks," transcript p. 2, https://unnaturalcauses.org/assets/uploads/file/UC_Transcript_2 .pdf.

30. *Being Serena,* season 1, episode 1, 19:30.

31. Fran Kritz, "A New Campaign to Reduce C-Sections Is Especially Critical for African-American Mothers and Babies," *California Health Report,* August 10, 2018, https://www.calhealthreport.org/2018/08/10/ new-campaign-reduce-c-sections-especially-critical-african-american -mothers-babies/.

32. *Being Serena,* season 1, episode 1, 17:00.

33. *Being Serena,* season 1, episode 2, 10:30.

34. Alondra Nelson, *Body and Soul: The Black Panther Party and the Fight against Medical Discrimination* (Minneapolis: University of Minnesota Press, 2013), 20.

35. Terry Kapsalis, "Mastering the Female Pelvis: Race and the Tools of Reproduction," in *Skin Deep, Spirit Strong: The Black Female Body in American Culture,* ed. Kimberly Wallace-Sanders, 263–300 (Ann Arbor: University of Michigan Press, 2002).

36. Deirdre Cooper Owens, *Medical Bondage: Race, Gender, and the Origins of American Gynecology* (Athens: University of Georgia Press, 2018).

37. Deborah Gray White, *Ar'n't I a Woman? Female Slaves in the Plantation South* (New York: W. W. Norton, 1985).

38. Chelsea Litchfield, Emma Cavanagh, Jaquelyn Osborne, and Ian Jones, "Social Media and the Politics of Gender, Race and Identity: The Case of Serena Williams," *European Journal for Sport and Society* 15, no. 2 (2018): 154–70.

39. Marc Peyser and Alison Samuels, "Venus and Serena against the World," *Newsweek,* August 24, 1998, 46.

40. For examples and analysis, see Delia D. Douglas, "'Dis' Qualified! Serena Williams and Brittney Griner: Black Female Athletes and the Politics of the Im/Possible," in *Relating Worlds of Racism: Dehumanisation, Belonging, and the Normativity of European Whiteness,* ed. Philomena Essed, Karen Farquharson, Kathryn Pillay, and Elisa Joy White, 329–55 (New York: Palgrave Macmillan, 2019), esp. 337.

41. Moya Bailey, "Misogynoir in Medical Media: On Caster Semenya and R. Kelly," *Catalyst: Feminism, Theory, Technoscience* 2, no. 2 (2016).

42. Delia D. Douglas, "Venus, Serena, and the Inconspicuous Consumption of Blackness: A Commentary on Surveillance, Race Talk, and New Racism(s)," *Journal of Black Studies* 43, no. 2 (2012): 127–45, esp. 133.

43. Janell Hobson, "The 'Batty' Politic: Toward an Aesthetic of the Black Female Body," *Hypatia* 18, no. 4 (2003): 87–105; see also James McKay and Helen Johnson, "Pornographic Eroticism and Sexual Grotesquerie in Representations of African American Sportswomen," *Social Identities* 14, no. 4 (2008): 491–504. The prominence of Baartman as an icon of nineteenth-century racial and sexual science can and should be problematized—see Zine Magubane, "Which Bodies Matter? Feminism, Poststructuralism, Race, and the Curious Theoretical Odyssey of the 'Hottentot Venus,'" *Gender and Society* 15, no. 6 (2001): 816–34—but the mobilization of the connection undoubtedly does powerful work in the twenty-first century.

44. For discussion, see Kristi Tredway, "The Performance of Blackness and Femininity in Postfeminist Times: Visualising Serena Williams within the Context of Corporate Globalisation," in *New Sporting Femininities: Embodied Politics in Postfeminist Times,* ed. Kim Toffoletti, Holly Thorpe, and Jessica Francombe-Webb, 63–85 (Cham, Switzerland: Palgrave Macmillan, 2018).

45. Steve Ginsburg, "Serena Finally Apologizes for Her Foot-Fault Rant," Reuters, September 14, 2009, https://www.reuters.com/article/us -tennis-open-serena/serena-finally-apologizes-for-foot-fault-rant-idUS TRE58D4JY20090914.

46. John William Devine, "Serena Williams's US Open Meltdown and Why On-Court Coaching Should Not Be Allowed," *Conversation,* September 10, 2018, https://theconversation.com/serena-williamss-us-open -meltdown-and-why-on-court-coaching-should-not-be-allowed-102925.

47. For a rich discussion of Williams's angry outburst and much more, see Raquel Kennon, "Uninhabitable Moments: The Symbol of Serena Williams, Rage and Rackets in Claudia Rankine's *Citizen: An American Lyric,*" in *Challenging Misrepresentations of Black Womanhood: Media, Literature and Theory,* vol. 1, ed. Marquita M. Gammage and Antwanisha Alameen-Shavers, 27–52 (London: Anthem Press, 2019).

48. See Therí A. Pickens, "The Verb Is No: Towards a Grammar of Black Women's Anger," *CLA Journal* 60, no. 1 (2016): 15–31, esp. her discussion of this element of Serena Williams's public persona (22).

49. Jaime Schultz, "Reading the Catsuit: Serena Williams and the Production of Blackness at the 2002 U.S. Open," *Journal of Sport and Social Issues* 29, no. 3 (2005): 338–57.

50. Roger Domeneghetti, "'The Other Side of the Net': (Re) Presentations of (Emphasised) Femininity during Wimbledon 2016," *Journal of Policy*

Research in Tourism, Leisure, and Events 10, no. 2 (2018): 151–63, esp. 159–60.

51. Quoted in Schultz, "Reading the Catsuit," 345.

52. Patricia Hill Collins, *Fighting Words: Black Women and the Search for Justice* (Minneapolis: University of Minnesota Press, 1998), 38.

53. Laurel Wamsley, "'One Must Respect the Game': French Open Bans Serena Williams' Catsuit," National Public Radio, August 24, 2018, https:// www.npr.org/2018/08/24/641549735/one-must-respect-the-game -french-open-bans-serena-williams-catsuit.

54. Serena Williams told reporters in a postmatch press conference, "I've had a lot of problems with my blood clots, God I don't know how many I've had in the past 12 months. I've been wearing pants in general a lot when I play so I can keep the blood circulation going." The comments were widely reported and discussed; see, e.g., Nadra Nittle, "The Serena Williams Catsuit Ban Shows That Tennis Can't Get Past Its Elitist Roots," *Vox,* August 28, 2018, https://www.vox.com/2018/8/28/17791518/ serena-williams-catsuit-ban-french-open-tennis-racist-sexist-country -club-sport; Luke Darby, "Serena Williams' Catsuit Is Banned from All Future French Opens," *GQ,* August 25, 2018.

55. Whitney McIntosh, "Serena Williams' French Open Catsuit Is for 'All the Moms Out There,'" *SBNation,* May 29, 2018, https://www.sbnation .com/tennis/2018/5/29/17406858/serena-williams-french-open -catsuit-pregnancy-recovery.

56. Ramona Coleman-Bell, "Droppin' It Like It's Hot: The Sporting Body of Serena Williams," in *Framing Celebrity: New Directions in Celebrity Culture,* ed. Su Holmes and Sean Redmond, 195–205 (New York: Routledge, 2006), esp. 196–97.

57. Schultz, "Reading the Catsuit," esp. 340.

58. For discussion, see Delia D. Douglas, "Venus, Serena, and the Women's Tennis Association: When and Where 'Race' Enters," *Sociology of Sport Journal* 22, no. 3 (2005): 255–81; see also Nancy E. Spencer, "Sister Act VI: Venus and Serena Williams at Indian Wells: 'Sincere Fictions' and White Racism," *Journal of Sport and Social Issues* 28, no. 2 (2004): 115–35.

59. Of course, their philanthropy itself could be seen as part of selling out to corporate capital—the narrative being individual success, and then supporting "giving back" over structural change. See Jayne O. Ifekwunigwe, "Venus and Serena Are 'Doing It' for Themselves," in *Marxism, Cultural Studies and Sport,* ed. Ben Carrington and Ian McDonald, 130–53 (Oxon, U.K.: Routledge, 2009).

60. *Being Serena,* season 1, episode 1, 19:40.
61. *Being Serena,* season 1, episode 2, 9:36. In the documentary, her agent, Jill Smoller, also reflects: "The enormity of everything was scary. But fortunately, because she advocated for herself, they ended up taking her in for a CAT scan, and they found the pulmonary embolism."
62. Audre Lorde, *A Burst of Light and Other Essays* (Ithaca, N.Y.: Firebrand Books, 1988), 130.

CONCLUSION

1. This was the subject of many news reports globally, e.g., in the *Guardian.* Nina Lakhani, "Detroit: Civil Rights Coalition Sues to Bar Water Shutoffs for Residents," *Guardian,* July 9, 2020.
2. See Larry R. Churchill, Nancy M. P. King, and Gail E. Henderson, "The Future of Bioethics: It Shouldn't Take a Pandemic," *Hasting Center Report* 50, no. 3 (2020): 54–56.
3. This assignment is also informed by those of other teachers, including those who taught me. It is particularly resonant with a popular exercise in courses in science and technology studies and related fields that involves mapping out diverse elements that come together in one particular object to explore the broader social world. See Joseph Dumit, "Writing the Implosion: Teaching the World One Thing at a Time," *Cultural Anthropology* 29, no. 2 (2014): 344–62. My template builds on that exercise, choosing a focal event rather than an object. Both exercises have a common goal: to sit longer with things and wake up to connections. As Dumit argues, "even if we read newspapers, watch cable news (CNN, BBC, or FOX), or follow and resend Facebook posts, the war-torn, poverty- and disease-stricken, unequal, unbearable world is tragic—but somehow tolerable. A problem shared, I would argue, by Haraway and Deleuze, is how to disrupt our own tolerance, how to see the intolerable in the everyday" (347).
4. These three levels of racism were laid out in the Introduction and are drawn from Jones, "Levels of Racism."
5. See Evelynn M. Hammonds and Susan M. Reverby, "Toward a Historically Informed Analysis of Racial Health Disparities since 1619," *American Journal of Public Health* 109, no. 10 (2019): 1348–49.
6. Camisha A. Russell makes this point while addressing her own field of bioethics, and it is no less relevant for many scholarly domains. Russell,

"Questions of Race in Bioethics: Deceit, Disregard, Disparity, and the Work of Decentering," *Philosophy Compass* 11, no. 1 (2016): 52.

7. For further discussion about authentic implementation, see Ashanté Reese and Hanna Garth, "Beyond the Parentheticals: The Practice of Being in Conversation," *gradfoodstudies* 6, no. 1 (2019), https://gradfood studies.org/2019/06/16/beyond-the-parentheticals/.

8. Although being intentional about citation in that way can be an interesting exercise, and open up space for engaging with more feminist voices, as Sara Ahmed demonstrated in her *Living a Feminist Life* (Durham, N.C.: Duke University Press, 2017), in which she cited no white men.

9. See https://www.sistersong.net/reproductive-justice.

10. See https://blacklivesmatter.com/category/chapters/.

11. See https://www.snap4freedom.org/home.

12. See https://www.charisbooksandmore.com/.

13. Jonathan M. Metzl and Helena Hansen, "Structural Competency: Theorizing a New Medical Engagement with Stigma and Inequality," *Social Science and Medicine* 103 (2014): 126–33.

14. Kim Krisberg, "Programs Work from within to Prevent Black Maternal Deaths: Workers Targeting Root Cause—Racism," *Nation's Health: A Publication of the American Public Health Association* 49, no. 6 (2019): 1–17.

15. Mary T. Bassett, "#BlackLivesMatter—a Challenge to the Medical and Public Health Communities," *New England Journal of Medicine* 372, no. 12 (2015): 1085–87.

16. Start by reading the organization's website: https://whitecoats4blacklives.org/.

17. "King Berates Medical Care Given Negroes," Associated Press, March 26, 1966. King's quote has been rendered in different ways and is itself a rich site of analysis; see Charlene Galarneau, "Getting King's Words Right," *Journal of Health Care for the Poor and Underserved* 29, no. 1 (2018): 5–8.

18. "Health is more than a medical matter" is a mantra of my current department, Global Health and Social Medicine at King's College London (https://blogs.kcl.ac.uk/ghsm/).

Index

Page numbers in italic refer to illustrations.

activism, 15; anti-police brutality, 114, 134; antiprison, 64, 70–72; environmental, 91–92, 174n22; gatekeeping, lack of, 114; peer-to-peer sharing, 114. *See also* Black Lives Matter; civil rights movement

African Americans, 4, 34, 44, 48, 67, 71, 82, 100, 130, 135–36; bodily suffering, 72; and citizenship, 59; Great Migration, 81; living donors, and risk, 75; medical providers, distrust of, 21–22, 40; Postal Service, 25–27; as second-class citizens, treatment of, 38; social control of, 46; suffering, as invisible, 37; treatment compliance, 29

African American studies, 12

Afrofuturism, 114, 182n60

age, 40, 140; of elders, 46, 51; and teens, 18, 95–97, 103; young ages, denial of care, impact of, 56; younger ages, and vulnerability to disease, 137

agency, 72–73, 129

Ahmed, Sara, 189n8

Alcaraz, Lalo, 108

Alexander, Amy, 40; whitewashing of terror, 37, 39

Alexander, Michelle, 46, 68, 111

Allen Park (Michigan), 173n14

All Lives Matter, 92

altruism, 72

Ambrose, Gerald, 173n16

American Civil Liberties Union (ACLU), 84

American College of Cardiology (ACC), 45–46

American Dream, 128

American Public Health Association, 67

Amuchie, Nnennaya, 103

Anand, Nikhil, 88, 89

anthrax attacks, 21–24, 26–28, 32–33, 35–37, 156n53; Black postal workers, 3, 5, 15–16, 134–35; class, focus on, 25; postal workers, as group and testing, 30; and skepticism, 29, 31; Tuskegee Syphilis Study, 152n2

anthropocentrism, 91

antibiotics, 32; misuse, concern about, 28

anti-Black racism, 4, 123, 147n5; Black people, impact on, 9

antiprison activism, 71, 72
antiracism: and racism, 18, 95–96
Appiah, Anthony, 75–76
Arbery, Ahmaud, 1, 133
Arkansas National Guard, 160n27
Association of Black Cardiologists, 46, 143
Atlanta (Georgia), 15, 121, 144, 183n13
Attack of the 50 Foot Woman (film), 108, *109*

Baartman, Saartjie, 126, 186n43
Bailey, Moya, 14, 126
Bailey, Zinzi, 9
Barbour, Haley, 61, 63–66, 73, 75
Barthes, Roland: reality effect, 113
Beal, Frances, 26
Becton, Dajerria, 18, 95–97, 102–4, 107–8, 110
belonging: imagined communities of, 53; play and, 99
Bell, Jimmy, 30
Benjamin, Ruha, 2, 22, 76–77, 107, 114; New Jim Crow, 111–12
Bennett, Jane, 90–91
Benton Harbor (Michigan), 173n14
bioethics, 17, 75–76, 188n6
biological citizenship, 12, 15, 17, 59, 61, 69–70, 72–73; prison activism, 71; as racialized, 65
biomedicine: and race, 6, 114, 130–31
biopolitics, 10–12, 15, 17, 45, 59, 72–73, 89, 93, 95, 165n73; infrastructure of cities, 58; as racialized, 80; and racism, 58; and surveillance, 96

biopower, 10–11; meaning of, 58
Black Church, 143; prisoners, advocacy for, 72
Black feminist theory, 150n24
Black Feminist Think Tank, 121
"Black Girl Song for Dajerria," 102
Black Lives Matter, 1, 13, 19, 91–92, 97, 99, 103, 106, 110, 114, 133–35, 137, 143, 151n33, 183n13
Blackness, 7, 13, 126; chronic disease, association with, 53
Black Panther (film), 128
Black Panther Party: health activism of, 71
Black patients: racialized framing of, 159n15
Black postal workers, 35, 37, 39, 41; antibiotics, concern about, 28
Black Radical Congress, 26
Black women, 118, 126, 129–30, 141, 144; C-sections, 124; as hypersurveilled, 117; maternal mortality rate, 19, 117, 119, 121–22, 124, 182n6; as sites of extraction, 125; stress, and premature births, 184n23; surgical sterilization, as "Mississippi appendectomies," 76; surveillance of, 127–28; "weathering" of, 123
Blanco, Kathleen, 48, 160n27
body-shaming, 102, 179n27
Brazil, 147n5
Bridges, Khiara, 123–24
Brock, James, *105*
Brown, Michael, 97, 99, 103–4
Brown, Ruth Nicole, 103
Bush, George W., 36, 40

Canada, 70
capitalism: and automation, 87; consumer, 69
Caplan, Arthur, 75
carcerality, 76–77
Casartelli, Sara, 174n22
Casebolt, Eric, 97, 102–3
Catholic liberation theology, 91–92
Centers for Disease Control and Prevention (CDC), 24–25, 28, 30, 32, 35–37, 52, 119, 122–23, 153n10, 156n50
Cerise, Fred, 50
Charis Books & More, 144
Charity Hospital, 55, 163n55; de facto segregation of, 54
Chernobyl (Ukraine), 69
Cho, Mildred K., 148n10
Christianity, 71–72, 170n62
chronic disease, 3, 11, 16, 44, 50–51, 54, 56–57, 93, 135, 142; and Blackness, 53; and modernity, 53
Chun, Wendy Hui Kyong, 104, 112, 114
Cipro, 22, 28–29, 153n6, 155n28
citizenship, 48–49, 66, 80, 87, 130; biological, 12; biopolitics, 12; Black people, 59; citizenship rights, 68–69; contestation over, 12; corporate, 89; femininity, denial of, 125; health, disparities in, 73; incomplete, 53; individual level of, 12–13; pharmaceuticals, 59; racialization of, 3, 59, 161; safe water, as basic right of, 88, 90
Civil Rights Act (1871), 66
civil rights movement, 13, 54, 100, 104, 106, 110, 137, 166n7; and photography, 114
Civil War, 65, 101
class: American Dream, 128; in Flint (Michigan), 81; and gender, 10–11, 128, 140; health disparities, 122; mass incarceration, 68; maternal health disparities, 122; postal workers, 25–27, 37, 41; privilege, 25; and race, 9–11, 27, 37, 41, 68, 122, 128, 140; and racism, 9–11; and segregation, 101. *See also* middle class; poverty
Clinton, Bill, 6
Cohen, Lawrence, 74
Cohen, Mitch, 28
Coleman, Beth, 112–14
Collins, Patricia Hill, 127–28
colonialism, 5, 82
Combs, Barbara Harris, 101
Coming Soon: Attack of the 14-Year-Old Black Girl! (cartoon), 108, *109*
Condit, Celeste M., 148n10
Cooper, Brittney, 103
coronavirus, 1, 133–34, 136–38, 145. *See also* COVID-19
corporate personhood, 12, 88
COVID-19, 1–2, 19, 133–35, 137, 144. *See also* coronavirus
criminal justice, 69, 74; racial inequality, perpetuating of, 65; as structurally racist, 68
critical race studies, 76–77
cultural bioethics, 75
Curseen, Joseph P., Jr., 15–16, 21, 23, 27–31, 36, 41, 154n13, 154n23
Cutter, Susan, 56

Daily Show, The (TV show), 107–8
Das, Veena, 40–41
Daschle, Tom, 22–23, 28, 35–36, 39
David, Richard, 124
Davis, Dána-Ain, 121–22
debt, 74, 82–85
deindustrialization, 81, 173n11
de Leeuw, Marc, 88
Deleuze, Gilles, 188n3
deprivation, 9, 69, 71–73, 95–96, 139
desegregation, 100, 104, 127
Detroit (Michigan), 84, 136, 173nn13–14
Detroit Water and Sewage Department, 79
Diallo, Amadou, 7
dialysis: incarceration, comparisons with, 68
digital archiving projects, 14
discard studies, 176n50
durability, 7, 149n12
drug laws: Black and poor, disenfranchising of, 46–47. *See also* War on Drugs
Dumit, Joseph, 188n3
Dumont, Dora M., 67

Earley, Darnell, 173n16
Ecorse (Michigan), 173n14
Egypt, 68
Ehlers, Nadine, 11, 76–77
Eighth Amendment, 66
emergency financial management, 84, 86, 173n14, 173n16, 174n23; in Black majority cities, 173n13; strategic racism, 174n31; subversion of democratic processes,

82–83; unequal access to power, role of, 85
environmental activism, 92
environmental justice, 3
environmental racism, 80; as slow violence, 92
epidemic disease: and poor, 177n54
Estelle v. Gamble, 66
eugenics, 58
Eurocentrism, 165n73
Evert, Chris, 126

Facebook, 2
family advocacy: and activism, 23, 31, 62
Farmer, Paul, 76, 177n54
Federal Emergency Management Agency (FEMA), 79–80
feminist activism, 15, 111, 119, 129, 144
feminist scholarship, 13–14, 87, 90, 102–3, 121, 126–27
Ferguson (Missouri), 97, 99
Fields, Barbara, 7
Fishman, Jennifer R., 75
fistula, 125
Fleisher, Ari, 36
Flint (Michigan), 172n3, 173n14; Black population of, 172n10; deindustrialization of, 173n11; General Motors, disinvestment in, 81–82, 91; infrastructure of, 91; lead, brain-damaging levels of, 79; politics of abandonment, 86; racialized biopolitics, 80; water crisis, 3, 11–12, 17–18, 48–49, 79, 82–85, 87–93, 96, 136, 138, 173n16, 174n22, 174n27; white flight, 81

Flint Lives Matter, 91–92, 177n54
Flint Sit-Down Strike, 81
Florida, 28, 43, 66–67, 97, 99
Floyd, George, 1, 133
Ford, Tanisha, 102
forensic care, 174n22
Foucault, Michel, 11–13, 17, 76–77,
    95–96; biopolitics, idea of, 45, 58,
    165n73; biopower, emergence of,
    10; "Society Must Be Defended"
    phrase, 172n8
Fox News, 110
France, 102

gender: body-shaming, 102; and
    class, 10–11, 128, 140; gendered
    space, control of, 102; medical
    case reports, 40; and race, 10–11,
    18, 75, 127–28, 140; and swim-
    suits, 102
General Motors (GM), 3, 17–18,
    79–80, 82, 84, 86–88, 91–92,
    136, 138; citizenship, privilege
    form of, 89; as corporate citizen-
    ship, 89; preferential treatment
    of, 81
genetics, 6, 72, 148n10
genocide, 73, 183n13
Georgia, 133
ghettoization, 111
global health charity, 17
Global Health Complex, 50
Global North, 52
Global South, 50, 52
Goodwin, Michele, 71
Gravlee, Clarence C., 148n10
Great Lakes Water Authority,
    84
Great Migration, 81

Hall, Wiley, 25
Hamdy, Sherine, 170n62; political
    etiology, 68
Hamer, Fannie Lou, 76
Hammer, Peter J., 174n31
Hammonds, Evelynn, 8, 34–35,
    147n4
Hamtramck (Michigan), 173n14
Haraway, Donna, 13–14, 188n3
Harris-Perry, Melissa, 12, 47, 59,
    151n33
Hartnell, Anna, 164n65
Hatch, Anthony "Tony" Ryan, 11,
    66, 76–77
HBO Sports, 124, 129
health: police violence, 95; segrega-
    tion, 95
health care, 1–3, 27; inadequacy of,
    68; past incarceration, deleterious
    impact on, 67; pharmaceuticals,
    44; prisoners, constitutional right
    to, 66; racial disparities in, 80
health inequality, 1, 57, 59
health insurance, 27, 33, 54–56,
    156n47. See also managed care;
    Medicaid; Medicare
Herbert, Bob, 63
Here's to Flint (documentary), 84
HIV/AIDS, 57, 70; anti-Black
    racism, 4
Holloway, Karla, 75
Hollywood Shuffle (film), 26
Honoré, Russel, 48
Houston (Texas), 55
Human Genome Project, 6
human politics, 15
Hunt, Linda M., 148n10
Hurricane Katrina, 3, 11–12,
    16–17, 43, 54, 93, 135, 143, 158n7,

161n32, 165n74; aftermath of, 59;
biopolitics of racism, as emblematic of, 58; chronic conditions, of
survivors, 55–56; chronic disease,
contributing to, 44; donations,
51–52; as humanitarian crisis,
50; impact of, 57–58; incomplete
citizenship, 53; infrastructure,
failure of, 58; looting during,
47–49; and marginalization, 45,
57; media coverage of, 47–48, 57;
pharmaceuticals, flow of, 44–45,
47, 49–52, 55–57; and refugees,
49–50; shoot-to-kill orders, 48;
victims of, and criminality, association with, 45–47, 49. *See also*
New Orleans
Hurricane Maria, 161n32
Hurricane Sandy, 161n32
Hutchison, Sikivu, 103
hydraulic citizenship, 88–89

images: advocacy for justice,
mobilizing of, 19, 104–7, 110,
137; social media, distributing
of, 18–19, 96, 102; of Serena
Williams, 127
imagined communities: and chronic
disease, 53. *See also* belonging
Inda, Jonathan Xavier, 72
India, 74
Institute of Medicine, 156n47
institutionalized racism, 8, 66, 85,
93, 111, 138–39, 142
International Monetary Fund
(IMF), 86
intersectional feminism, 15, 90, 144
intersectionality, 150n24; and class,
10
Iraq, 48, 160n27

Irving, Shalon, 122–23
Islam, 170n62
Island of Flowers (short film), 86

Japan, 170n62
Jim Crow, 54, 68, 76, 111
Johns Hopkins Center for Civilian
Biodefense Studies, 30–31
Jones, Camara, 8, 85, 184n26
Jones, Mimi, *105*
Jones, Tatiana, 97

Kahn, Jonathan, 182n61
Kaiser Permanente, 33; lawsuit
against, 32, 156n52
Karegnondi Water Authority, 79,
83
Kentucky, 133
King, Martin Luther, Jr., 144–45,
166n7
kinship, 70, 112; and care, 71–72;
genetic ties, 72
knowledge: as insufficient to drive
action, 87; power, as inseparable,
13, 71, 140
Koenig, Barbara, 148n10
Koplan, Jeffrey, 29–30, 35
Krieger, Nancy, 10, 184n26
Krupar, Shiloh, 11, 76–77

Lacks, Henrietta, 147n7; HeLa cell
line from, 5
Lake Huron, 79
Latin America, 9, 155n28
Lee, Sandra Soo-Jin, 148n10
lesbians, 15, 129
liberatory imagination, 19, 96,
107
lifeboat ethics, 137
Lincoln Park (Michigan), 173n14

Lock, Margaret, 170n62
London (England), 15, 126, 133, 179n27
Lorde, Audre, 111, 129–30
Louisiana, 16, 43
Luhrmann, Tanya, 33–34
Lumumba, Chokwe, 62–63

MacLeod, Janine, 175n39
Malcolm X Grassroots Movement, 62, 143
Mamo, Laura, 75
managed care: paternalist dyad, contrast with, 33–34; snap judgments, 34
Margolis, Jane, 99
Marshall, Patricia, 148n10
Martin, Trayvon, 97, 99
Martucci, Jessica, 71
Masquelier, Adeline, 49
mass incarceration, 3, 17, 59, 68–69, 71–72, 75, 111, 136, 168n41; carceral, as term, 77; as carceral institution, 76; excessive sentencing, 63; public health consequences of, 67; as race-making institution, 76; racialized system of, 76; as racist institution, 61; structural violence of, 77
materiality: of images, 110; and the integrity of bodies versus machines, 18, 80, 89; material conditions and inequality, 45, 85, 89, 113; and semiotics, 13, 87, 102, 113
McClinton, Claire, 84
M'charek, Amade, 174n22
McKinney (Texas), 18, 95–97, 104, 106; demographics of, 100–101;

segregation in, 101; and white flight, 100
McKinney pool incident, 97, 99, 106, 137, 180n39; cell phone video, 107–8, 110; as "Jim Crow State of Mind," 101; race as technology, 112; as racial terrorism, 102–3; as sexual terrorism, 102–3
McMillan Cottom, Tressie, 122
Medicaid, 55, 66–67
medical care, 3, 6, 8, 22, 68, 138; chemical castration, 74; and reduced sentences, 74; denial of, 22, 66, 143. *See also* health care
medical ethics, 75–76. *See also* bioethics
medicalization, 124
Medicare, 55–56, 66
metabolic syndrome, 11
Mexico, 81
Michigan, 15, 81–83, 86, 173n13, 177n54; African American residents in, 173n14
Michigan National Guard, 79–80
middle class, 27–28, 81, 96, 101, 122, 155n23
miscegenation, 102
Miss America pageant, 102
Mississippi, 17, 43, 63–64, 66–67, 71–72
MondoHomo queer music and arts festival, 144
Monson Motor Lodge, *105, 106*
Moore, Michael, 81
Morris, Thomas L., Jr., 15–16, 21, 23–24, 27–30, 32, 36, 41, 154n13, 156n52
Mumbai (India), 88–89
Murphy, Michelle, 90

National Association for the Advancement of Colored People (NAACP), 62

National Guard, 58; at Superdome, 46–47, 51

National Health Service (NHS), 54

National Postal Museum, 154n16

Native Americans, 9, 40–41

Nazi Germany, 58

Nelson, Alondra, 71, 114, 124–25, 182n60

Nelson, Jill, 41

New Jim Crow, The (Alexander), 68, 111

New Orleans (Louisiana), 16, 57, 59, 135; branding of, 164n65; chronic disease, 44, 50; Convention Center, 44; flooding of, 43–45; infrastructure, failure of, 58; looting, 47; National Guard in, 46, 51; public hospital system, reliance on, 54; safety net, 55; social order, restoration of, 47; Superdome, 44–47, 49; as unequal city, 43; as war zone, 48–49. *See also* Hurricane Katrina

New South, 100

New York, 28, 37–38, 161n32

Nguyen, Vinh-Kim, 70

Nixon, Rob, 92–93; slow violence, 148n8

North America, 170n62

Obama, Barack, 79–80, 84–85, 88

Obamacare, 85

Ohanian, Alexis, 129

organ donation, 61, 64–65, 68–69, 71, 73, 170n62; and altruism, 72; Christian trope of, 72; and debt, 74; prison release, in exchange for, 75

Oxfam, 50

Parks, Rosa, 110

Parvin, Nassim, 14

Peoples, Whitney, 14

Petryna, Adriana, 69–71

pharmaceuticalization, 52

pharmaceuticals, 16–17, 44–45, 49–52; and citizenship, 59; disruption of, 47, 54–57; race based, 182n61; racialized concern about misuse, 28

Phoenix (Arizona), 83

police brutality, 1, 3, 18, 104; police uniform, as technology of racial terrorism, 102; and segregation, 137

police violence, 96, 99, 104, 134–35, 145, 178n4; amateur videos of, 113–14; and health, 95

policing, 1–2, 48, 95, 111; segregation, enforcing of, 18

pollution, 8, 90

Pontiac (Michigan), 173n14

Porto Alegre (Brazil), 86

posthumanist feminism, 90

Potter, John E. "Jack," 29–30, 36, 39

poverty, 19, 27; COVID-19, impact of, 135; dispossession, 85; environmental racism, 85; Hurricane Katrina, impact of, 43, 47, 49–50, 52–53, 55–57; and incarceration, 67–70, 74; poor, preferential option for, 91, 177nn54–55

prenatal care, 117; and race, 57

Prime, Markus, 108, 181n44

Prince Georges County (Maryland), 27
prison system, 64, 142, 145; abolition, calls for, 136; activism, as biological citizenship project, 71; biological control, 61; Black church, advocacy for, 72; and citizenship, 70, 73, 136; coronavirus outbreaks, 136; debt relationship of, 74; exclusion from society, 76; flawed medical care, 67–68; health disparities, 67; prison population, growth of, 67; racial inequality, contribution to, 77; as racialized, 76; rehabilitate, failure to, 76; release, in exchange for kidney donation, ethical problem of, 75; release from, as moneysaving device, 66; right to health care, 66–67, 70; slavery, rooted in, 65
public space, 101; and race, 104
Puerto Rico, 161n32

queer, 15, 144

race, 72, 77, 96, 110, 115; ambiguity of, 7; and biomedicine, 6, 114, 130–31; and class, 10–11, 41, 128; as concept, 7; durability of, 7; and gender, 18, 75, 127–28; in medical histories, 40; and medicine, 157n67; ontology of, 6; and poverty, 57; public space, 104; racial capitalism, 86; racial identities, as social processes, 7; racialized bodies, as disposable, 87; racial profiling, in health care, 29, 34–35; racial segregation, 111; racial terrorism, 102–3;

self-identified, 7; snap judgments, 7; as technology, 15, 19, 97, 102, 112–14; as visual, 8
racial inequality, 46, 113, 139; and surveillance, 77
racialization: of infectious disease, 163; partial citizenship, 3, 59, 161
racial justice, 48, 106–7, 143
racism, 2, 5, 10, 26, 39–41, 72, 82, 91, 106, 110, 126, 129, 142, 165n73, 188n4; accumulated insults, 184n26; and antiracism, 18, 95–96; and biopolitics, 58; and class, 9; and health, 114–15; health, impact on, 8, 21; in health care, 3–4, 144; health disparities, 8–9, 137–38; impact of, 6, 8; institutionalized, 8; internalized, 8; levels of, 8; personally mediated, 8; in science and technology studies, 7; as social practice, 6–7; and swimming pools, 101; visual media, 106, 111–12
Rasco, Evelyn, 62
Raynor, Clarence, 35
Reconstruction, 65–66
recreational spaces: as contested, 100. *See also* swimming pools
Red Cross, 47, 71
refugees, 50; international laws, 53; as sympathetic figures, 50; as term, 49; vulnerability of, 53
reproductive justice, 3, 19, 117, 119–22, 131, 137, 143
Richmond, Leroy, 23, 29, 31–33, 38, 40–41
Ridge, Tom, 25
Roberts, Dorothy, 120–21
Robinson, Whitney, 121

Roger and Me (film), 81, 85–86, 173n11
Rose, Nikolas, 69–71
Ross, Loretta, 121
Russell, Camisha A., 188n6

Sankar, Pamela, 148n10
Satcher, David, 36
Saxton, Gail, 38
#SayHerName, 110–11
Schwartz, Robert S., 157n67
science and technology studies (STS), 13–14, 75, 114, 188n3; nonhuman, interest in, 89–90; posthuman, 89; racism in, 7
Scott, Alicia Richmond, 31–32
Scott, Gladys, 3, 11–12, 17, 62, 67, 69–70, 73–74, 76, 136, 143; biopolitics, 72; and Christianity, 71–72; conditional release of, 63, 65–66, 75; kidney donation, 61, 63, 68, 71–72, 75; life sentence, suspension of, 61, 63–64; personhood of, 75
Scott, Jamie, 3, 11–12, 17, 69–70, 73–74, 76, 136, 143; biopolitics, 72; and Christianity, 71–72; conditional release of, 65–66, 75; kidney failure, 62, 68; life sentence, suspension of, 61, 63–64; medical maltreatment of, 62–63, 67–68; personhood of, 75
segregation, 1, 10, 139, 144–45; and health, 95; police enforcement of, 18, 137; structural racism, fundamental element of, 99; swimming pools, 101–2, 104; transgression of space, reaction to, 101
Semenya, Caster, 126
September 11 attacks, 2, 5, 22, 37–38, 40–41, 56, 59, 134–35, 165n74; "all in this together," as lie, 6, 16
settler colonies, 9, 147n5, 178n13
sexuality, 10, 71, 126–27, 140
sexual terrorism, 102–3
Sharpe, Christina, 123
Shim, Janet, 10–11
Simon, Susan Whyte, 32–33
Sims, Marion, 125
SisterSong Women of Color Reproductive Justice Collective, 121, 143; Trust Black Women project, 183n13
Skloot, Rebecca, 147n7
Slaughter, Vanessa, 25
slavery, 5, 34, 40–41, 65–66, 73, 111
Smith, Erna, 37–38
Smith, Roger, 81
Smithsonian Institution, 154n16
Smoller, Jill, 188n61
Snyder, Rick, 79–80
social injustices: template for analysis, 138–42
social media, 2, 18–19, 110, 130–31, 133–34, 137
Social Text (journal), 182n60
"Society Must Be Defended" (Foucault), 17, 45, 58
Solnit, Rebecca, 47
Solutions Not Punishment, 144
sousveillance, 178n4
South Africa, 147n5
South Asia, 155n28
South Carolina, 73–74
sovereignty, 58
Spicer, Paul, 148n10
Sports Illustrated (magazine): swimsuit issue, 179n25

St. Augustine (Florida), 104, *105, 106,* 110
Stewart, Jon, 108
Strategic National Stockpile, 51
strategic racism, 174n31
structural inequality, 134
structural racism, 75, 174n31; and segregation, 99. *See also* institutionalized racism
structural violence, 135
suburbs, 18, 81, 104, 113; homeowner association-controlled pools, 100; manufacturing, suburbanization of, 88; racialization of, 100. *See also* swimming pools
surveillance, 12; and biopolitics, 96; of Black bodies, 101; racial inequality, contributing to, 77; of urban space, 76
swimming pools, 113, 115, 178n13; as contested space, 100; racialized control of space in, 102; racism, enactment of, 101; and segregation, 101, 104, 178n13; segregation of, by sex, 102; as sites of exclusion, 99; "swim-in," 104, 106, 110; white families, domain of, 100
swimsuits, 96; bikinis, as freedom, 102, 179n27; body-shaming, 102, 179n27; as technologies of gender, 102; women's bodies, control over, 102

Taylor, Breonna, 1, 133
tennis, 128; white elite space of, 126, 129
terrorism, 3, 37, 135; rhetorics of, 56; sexual, 102–3
therapeutic citizenship, 61, 70, 72

Tierney, Kathleen, 47–48, 165n74
Towns, Armond R., 111
transplant medicine: and kinship, 71
Truth, Sojourner, 125
Tulane University Health Sciences Center, 56
Turkle, Sherry, 28–29
Tuskegee Syphilis Study, 5, 21–22, 34, 147n7, 152nn3–4; ethical violations of, 76

United Auto Workers (UAW), 81
United Kingdom, 1, 54
United States, 1, 5, 7–8, 16, 37, 40–41, 46, 48, 50, 52–54, 69, 75, 77, 80, 88, 89–91, 95, 117, 139, 141–42, 162n43; biological citizenship in, 70, 72–73; biopolitics, 73; care, unequal access to, 61; citizenship, racialization of, 3; criminal justice, 74; C-sections in, 124; double standards of life in, 39; health care, right to, 66; health care system, inadequacy of, 70, 135; health inequality in, 57; HIV/AIDS epidemic in, 4; incarceration rate, 65; organ donation, 71; public pools in, 99–100; race and class, as linked, 9–10; racial genocide, founding on, 73; racial health disparities in, 2–3; as settler colony, 9; social support systems, failures of, 56; U.S. South, 15, 57, 65–66, 81, 100, 151n33
urban space: control of, 76; race and class segregation in, 100, 104; riots in, 49; unequal infrastructures, 1, 59, 93, 100

U.S. Postal Service, 32, 39, 153n10, 156n50; African American employees of, 154n16; racial character of, 25–27, 29

van Wichelen, Sonja, 88
vigilante violence, 2, 99, 134–35, 145
Vrecko, Scott, 74
vulnerability, 1, 16, 18, 23, 44, 57, 95, 104; of Black lives, 92, 137; of refugees, 53; as structure, 6

Wacquant, Loïc, 76
Walks, Ivan, 28
War on Drugs, 68–69; color blindness, 46; racial control, as central to, 46
Washington, D.C., 22, 26–27, 37, 39
weathering, 123, 137
West Africa, 70, 155n28
West Jefferson Medical Center, 54
White Coats for Black Lives, 144
white flight, 81, 100
white supremacy, 104
Wiley, Ralph, 26–27
Williams, Anthony, 26, 36–37
Williams, Jessica, 107, *107,* 108

Williams, Serena, 3, 10, 119, *120,* 121–23, 125, 129–30, *130,* 131, 137; blood clots, problems with, 118, 128, 187n54; body, surveillance of, 127; catsuits, 127–28; as crossover celebrity, 117; C-section, 118, 124; dehumanization of, 12, 117; expression of anger, criticism for, 127; femininity, denial of, 126; hypervisibility of, 12, 117, 127; invisibility of, 127; misogyny, 126; parodying of, 126–27; pulmonary embolism, 118, 188n61; and racism, 126; and sexuality, 126
Williams, Sherri, 111
Williams, Venus, 126, 128–29
Winner, Langdon, 177n3
Women's Tennis Association (WTA), 128
Working Group on Race and Racism in Contemporary Biomedicine, 121
World Bank, 86
World Health Organization (WHO): health, definition of, 3
World War II, 86
Wozniacki, Caroline, 126–27

Anne Pollock is professor of global health and social medicine at King's College London. She is author of *Medicating Race: Heart Disease and Durable Preoccupations with Difference* and *Synthesizing Hope: Matter, Knowledge, and Place in South African Drug Discovery.*